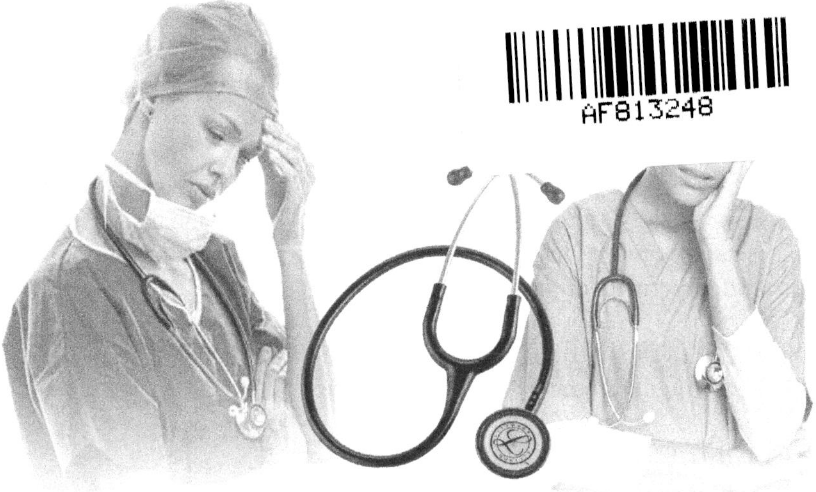

A Mindfulness Stress Reduction Program to Decrease Burnout in

NURSES AND CAREGIVERS

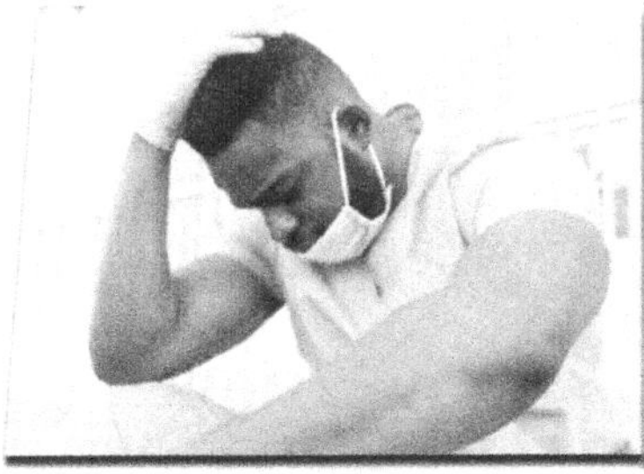

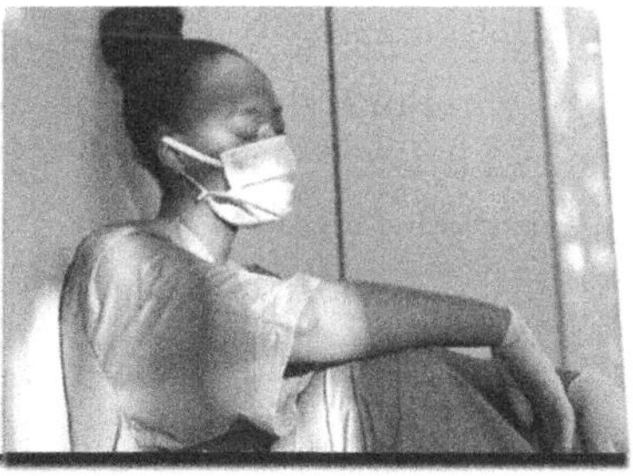

Dr. LaTarsha Bilal-Edwards
DNP, APRN, PMHNP-BC

Contact the Author: latarshae@yahoo.com

Author: Dr. LaTarsha Bilal-Edwards, DNP, APRN, PMHNP-BC
Publisher: Kingdom News Publication Services, LLC.

DISCLAIMER

All the material contained in this book is provided for educational and informational purposes only. No responsibility can be taken for any results or outcomes resulting from the use of this material.

While every attempt has been made to provide information that is both accurate and effective, the author does not assume any responsibility for the accuracy or use/misuse of this information.

Printed in the United States of America.
ISBN 978-1955127110

Library of Congress Control Number: 2022903865

Library of Congress
US Programs, Law, and Literature Division
Cataloging in Publication Program
101 Independence Avenue, S.E.
Washington, DC 20540-4283

KINGDOM NEWS TODAY
Publication Services, LLC

ACKNOWLEDGEMENTS

I would like to take a moment to thank God for the completion of this project and book. It is a labor of love. I would like to acknowledge, my mentors, instructors and family members for encouraging me to complete this project. I would like to give a special thank you to Apostle J.P. Smith for encouraging me to publish this book to help encourage and implement mindfulness to not only nurses but people who are caregivers.

PREFACE

This book is designed and compounded with evidence-based practice to help nurses learn and implement mindfulness to help decrease burnout in a nursing home environment and can be used in other healthcare environments as well. Caregivers can also use this book as a manual to decrease burnout. During this pandemic burnout in nurses are at a significantly high rate. I pray this book open your mind to help decrease stress and have a balanced life.

Sincerely,

Dr. LaTarsha Bilal-Edwards
DNP, APRN, PMHNP-BC

TABLE OF CONTENTS

ABSTRACT

The purpose of this systems-change project is to implement a stress management and health promotion program in Alzheimer's type units to decrease the perception of stress and burnout in psychiatric-mental health nurses who provide direct care to individuals in secured units. This systems-change project will implement mindfulness techniques as an effective tool for reducing the perception of stress and burnout. These mindfulness-based stress reduction and burnout prevention program will be implemented into staff development programs for nurses who work in locked units and psychiatric units in the community. Mindfulness-based stress reduction is an effective tool to support nurses psychologically and to improve work satisfaction.

Behavioral and psychological symptoms of dementia often lead to admission into long-term care facilities or to nursing home placement. High levels of stress and burnout are a significant problem for registered nurses (RNs) in long-term care. RNs who care for this population are at increased risk for burnout. The results of this program will indicate whether implementing a stress management and health promotion program using mindfulness-based interventions decreases stress and burnout in psychiatric nurses who work in Alzheimer's type dementia units.

This book will also help Doctoral Nursing Practice students develop their program by reading the methodology section in Chapter 3.

LIST OF TABLES

Table

CHAPTER I

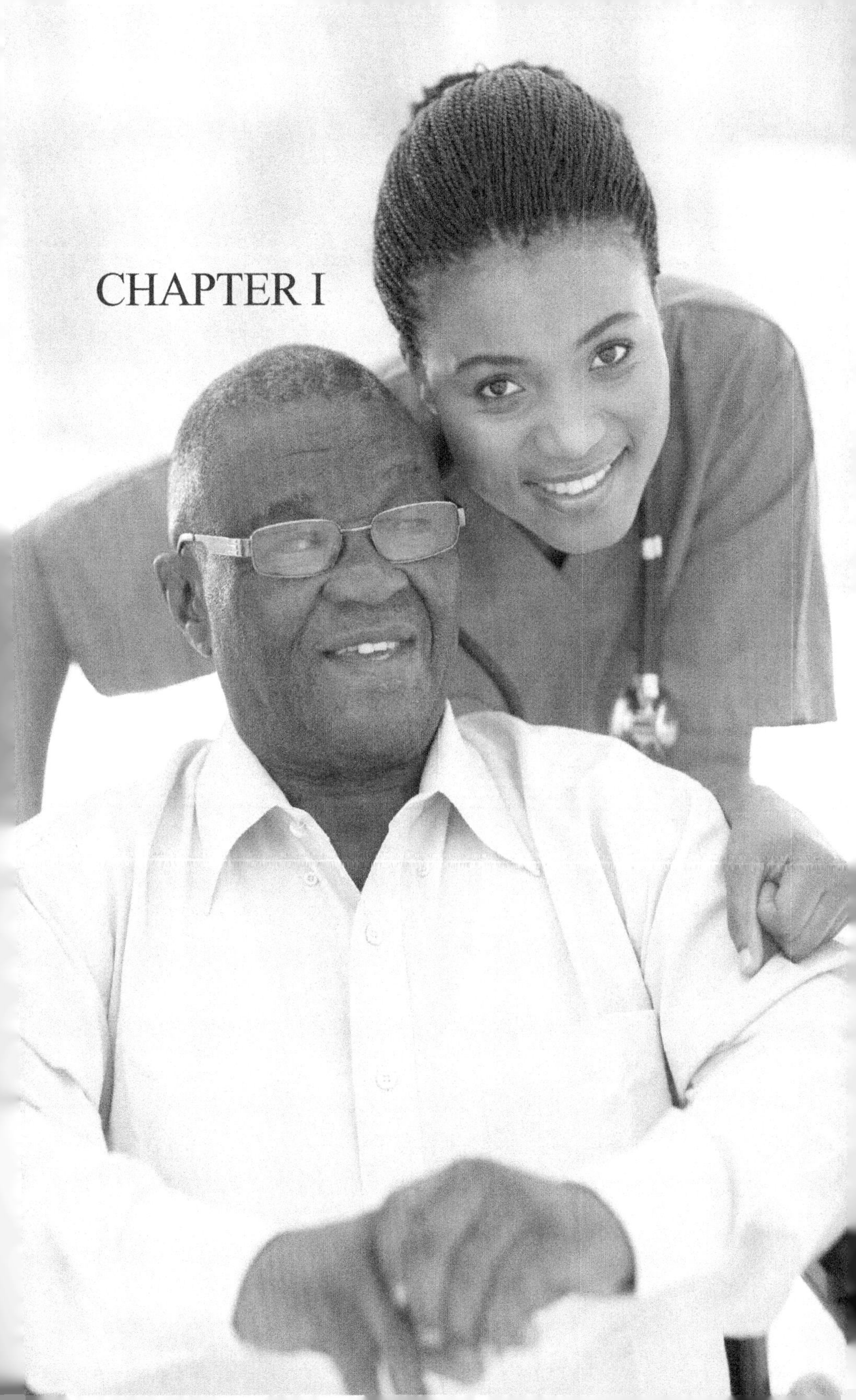

INTRODUCTION

Nursing is a profession that looks at individuals holistically. As caregivers, nurses must care for themselves in order to give fully to those they serve. Unmanaged stress can adversely affect the caring process. Nurses who leave the profession because they report feelings of exhaustion say they are unable to deliver quality of care to patients. Management of stress is a tool that is invaluable to the profession of nursing.

Work-related stress is a widespread problem and has shown to be costly to both individuals and organizations (Stanks, 2005). A review of literature identified that occupational stress cost U.S. economy 300 billion a year (Werner and Desimone, 2009). Related personal dysfunction includes physical exhaustion, insomnia, substance abuse, and interpersonal problems (Baba, Galperin, & Lituchy, 1999; Farrington, 1995). Greater organizational expenditures attributed to increased absenteeism, tardiness, staff turnover, low morale, decreased productivity and job satisfaction, and court-ordered compensation (Firth & Britton, 1989; Wheeler & Riding, 1994). Studies have demonstrated that the perception of burnout can jeopardize the professional's ability to provide high-quality care to patients (Coffey, 1999; Fagin et al., 1996; Jenkins & Elliott, 2004; Kilfedder, Power, & Wells, 2001).

According to AbuAlRub (2004), Balevre (2001), and Hall (2004), the nursing profession is a highly stressful occupation. When an individual experiences stress over an extended period in combination with ineffective coping, it can also lead to burnout (Maslach & Leiter, 1997). Burnout results in emotional exhaustion, reduced efficacy, and lower feelings of accomplishment (George, 2005). According to Maslach, Jackson, and Leiter (1996), burnout is "a syndrome of emotional exhaustion, depersonalization, and reduction of personal accomplishment that can occur among individuals who work with people in some capacity." However, George (2005) reported that as use of positive coping mechanisms increased, feelings of depression and anxiety decreased, and an increase in productive work was seen. Implementation of mindfulness-based stress reduction (MBSR) interventions will improve positive coping mechanisms, decrease the perception of stress and burnout, and improve quality of care and quality of life for dementia patients in locked units. MBSR interventions are effective in reducing stress and promoting well-being in clinical and non-clinical fields (Cohen-Katz et al., 2005; Gold et al., 2010; Penque, 2009; Shapiro, Astin, Bishop, & Cordova, 2005). Mindfulness training involves cultivating the ability to be aware of one's current thoughts, feelings, bodily sensations, and kindness and understanding. Mindfulness may improve patient care through patient safety, satisfaction, and quality of outcomes.

Mindfulness-Based Stress Reduction Program

Mindfulness-based stress reduction (MBSR) is a health care program that includes class instruction and practice of mindfulness techniques, meditation, and Hatha yoga designed to promote physical and psychological well-being (Kabat-Zinn, 1990). The MBSR program lasts eight weeks and is taught for 2.5 hours per week (Cohen-Katz, Wiley, Capuano, Baker, & Shapiro, 2004). The effectiveness of the MBSR program is supported in the literature for stress reduction.

The MBSR program's benefits have been documented in research studies for patients and include decrease in anxiety, pain, and depression as well as improved medical treatment and interventions (Epstein, 2003; Gross et al., 2004; Kabat-Zinn et al., 1992).

MBSR is a tool that can assist psychiatric RNs caring for patients with Alzheimer's type dementia in managing the perception of work stress and improving patient outcomes. Health professionals have conducted less than a dozen studies on the use of MBSR, and only two trials have focused exclusively on nurses and nursing assistants (Cohen-Katz et al., 2004; Mackenzie, Poulin, & Seidman-Carlson, 2006). Further studies are needed to narrow the gap in knowledge in the research of the MBSR program and its implementation for psychiatric nurses who work in Alzheimer's type dementia locked units.

Purpose of the Program

The purpose of this systems-change project is to implement a stress management and health promotion program using mindfulness interventions to decrease the perception of occupational stress and burnout in psychiatric-mental health nurses who provide direct care in psychiatric units to patients with Alzheimer's type dementia. Improving coping skills of RNs providing this type of care will reduce the perception occupational stress and burnout. Placing a mindfulness-based stress reduction and health promotion program in psychiatric Alzheimer's type dementia units would be a good systems change in practice to decrease the perception of occupational stress and burnout in psychiatric nurses. This data will propose a clinical change practice initiative. A program that I will recommend in orientation and presented yearly through the educational development program in nursing homes and hospitals to improve the emotional state of nurses to improve quality of care and patient outcomes in psychiatric units.

The PICOT question in this program indicates the (population) as the nurses, the (intervention) will be the implementation of a mindfulness program, (compared) to not implementing the mindfulness program; decrease the perception of stress and burnout which is the (outcome) over a four week period (time frame).

Needs Assessment

This program will provide a method of decreasing the perception of stress and burnout, specifically in nurses who work in psychiatric dementia-type units, to better understand nurses and formulate better polices and guidelines to meet their needs in stress reduction. The findings will add to the current body of knowledge pertaining to stress, coping, and burnout experienced by nurses who work in psychiatry. The findings can also provide these nurses with a better understanding the perception of occupational stressors, burnout, and coping mechanisms. This data will propose a clinical change practice initiative. A program that I will recommend in orientation and will be implemented through the staff development educational program in nursing homes and hospitals to improve the emotional health of nurses, increasing quality of care and improving patient outcomes.

Statement of the Problem

Psychiatric-mental health nurses working in locked units provide care for a patient population that requires increased observation and complex treatment modalities. This exposes psychiatric nurses to a variety of difficult and unique work-related stressors. Research has demonstrated that nurses working in other areas of psychiatry experience a significant level of stress. This program will examine the perception of stress and burnout in psychiatric nurses who work in locked units, their coping strategies, and the effectiveness of a mindfulness-based intervention program to decrease the perception of stress in RNs working in Alzheimer's type dementia units.

The researcher will address the following PICOT question in the program:

1. Will implementing a mindfulness-based stress reduction and health promotion intervention administered over a four-week period decrease the perception of stress and burnout of psychiatric nurses who care for patients with Alzheimer's type dementia compared to those who do not use this program.

Alzheimer's Type Dementia and Characteristics of the Disease Process

Dementia is a degenerative brain-based disease that is chronic and progresses into cognitive decline. Cognitive decline is a condition in which a person has a problem with memory, language, or another essential cognitive function, serious enough to be noticeable to others and to show up on test (Alzheimer's Association, 2007). Alzheimer's, which is the largest form of dementia, is a degeneration process that progresses through three stages: early, middle, and late. In early Alzheimer's a cognitive decline is seen in memory but does not affect activities of daily living (Alzheimer's Association, 2007). In early stages, clear symptoms include forgetfulness in several areas such as forgetfulness of recent events and impaired ability to perform challenging mental tasks, for instance, counting numbers from 100 backwards and subtracting in seven sequences. Other symptoms include greater difficulty performing complex tasks, such as planning dinner for guests, paying bills or managing finances, and forgetfulness about one's own personal history and becoming moody or withdrawn, especially in socially or mentally challenging situations.

In moderate Alzheimer's type dementia over an eight-to-ten-year span, a gradual increase in functional dependence and loss of ability to manage aspects of life such as shopping, managing financial responsibilities, and driving occurs (Alzheimer's Association, 2007). Gaps in memory and thinking are noticeable, and individuals begin to need help with day-to-day activities. Some symptoms of the middle stage of Alzheimer's type dementia include being unable to recall own address or phone number or high school or college from which the person graduated. In the middle stage of the disease, the person becomes more confused about where he or she is or what day it is and needs help choosing proper clothing for the season or the occasion while still remembering significant details about themselves and their family and still requiring no assistance with eating or using the toilet (Alzheimer's Association, 2012).

Eventually, in the late stages of Alzheimer's type dementia, grooming, toileting, dressing, and eating become impaired (Alzheimer's Association, 2007). The person loses awareness of recent experiences as well as of his or her surroundings; the person remembers his or her own name but has difficulty with personal history. In the late stages of this disease, the person is unable to distinguish familiar and unfamiliar faces and has trouble remembering the name of a spouse or caregiver. The person will need help putting on clothes and shoes and assistance with activities of daily living. In late-stage dementia, the patient may experience major personality and behavioral changes, including suspiciousness and delusions (such as believing the caregiver is an imposter or someone else) (Alzheimer's Association, 2012).

In the final, or end, stage of the disease, individuals may not be able to say words, toilet themselves, or help with their daily personal care, including eating. They lose the ability to respond to their environment or to carry on a conversation; lose the ability to ambulate and control muscle reflexes; swallowing also becomes impaired (Alzheimer's Association, 2012).

Dementia prevalence increases dramatically with age. The prevalence of dementia is 3–11% in people older than 65 and 25–47% in people older than 85 (USPSTF, 2003). As the disease progresses, professional nursing staff is needed to provide care for those affected with dementia. According to Alzheimer's Association

(2007), it was estimated that the number of those afflicted with Alzheimer's type dementia (which is the largest form of dementia) would increase from 454,000 new cases a year by 2010 to 615,000 new cases a year by 2030 and to 959,000 new cases a year by 2050. The increasing prevalence of dementia and the associated increase in dementia-related health care costs have prompted a call for nurses and long-term care facilities. There is a need for cost-effective interventions to increase nurses' skills and to provide safe, quality care to patients with Alzheimer's type dementia in long-term settings.

In long-term care facilities, nurses play a prominent role in caregiving by performing assessment, administering medication, and documenting the patient's response to medication. The need for long-term care services increases if a person cannot perform activities such as dressing, bathing, shopping, and managing money (Alzheimer's Association, 2013). "State and federal Medicaid spending for nursing home care for people with Alzheimer's and other dementias were estimated in 2013, 142 billion.

Federal and state government governments combined will spend an estimated $35 billion under the Medicaid program. Government spending represents 70 percent of the total costs of caring for those with Alzheimer's. "In 2050, Medicare will spend a project $627 billion caring for people with Alzheimer's disease – an increase of nearly 600 percent between 2010 and 2050." (Alzheimer's Association, 2013)." Medicaid spending on people with Alzheimer's will increase nearly 400 percent between 2010 and 2050, as cost will reach $178 billion in 2050." (Alzheimer's Association, 2013).

According to a study conducted by Kennedy (2005), RNs had more stress and burnout than any other level of nursing; but all nursing staff levels, while performing job duties, showed significant correlation between stress and inadequate preparation to meet the emotional needs of the patients.

If stress is not managed, it may lead to occupational burnout. Occupational burnout refers to the process of emotional exhaustion, decreased or reduced efficacy, and negative attitudes towards work and environment. Nurses experiencing high levels of burnout often plan to leave their current jobs or the nursing profession altogether (Vahey, Aiken, Sloane, Clarke, & Vargas, 2004). Burnout has also become a popular research topic in health care because of its impact on nurse retention and patient outcomes (Aiken, Clarke, Sloane, Sochalski, & Silber, 2002). It is important to find ways of helping nurses cope more effectively with the emotional demands of their work. Studies have shown that positive coping strategies protect against psychological distress, and that nurses are more likely to use positive coping strategies, especially in nursing home settings (Evers, Tomic, & Brouwers, 2002).

Patients of nurses suffering from burnout experience significantly lower levels of satisfaction with their care (Vahey et al., 2004). Mental health nurses are particularly vulnerable due to a lack of community support, low staffing levels, stigma, and client pressures including the risk of violence. The prevalence of burnout among mental health nurses has reached as high as 59.2%; therefore, the need for intervention is imperative (Imai, Nakao, Tsuchiya, Kuroda, & Katoh, 2004). Burnout causes significant problems related to care provision in mental health care settings because nurses suffering from burnout may become cynical, lose respect or concern for their patients, and become dehumanized to their patients' needs (Berling, 2001). In addition, the increasing number of mental health patients compared to the decreasing number of beds and qualified staff means that mental health nurses are spending less time per patient thus providing a reduced level of care (De Carlo, 2013).

Therefore, implementing a mindfulness-based stress reduction and health promotion program for RNs taking care of Alzheimer's type dementia patients is imperative in order to assure high quality of care for patients in long-term care facilities. It is possible through evidence-based practice interventions that have the potential to improve service provision.

The purpose of this mindfulness-based stress reduction and health promotion program is to decrease stress and burnout in psychiatric nurses who care for Alzheimer's type dementia patients. The implementation of this program will improve quality of care and quality of life for Alzheimer's type dementia patients. Decreasing stress will improve the caring process that is given by RNs. This program will improve the health care delivery system of this population.

According to Jalowiec, Murphy, and Powers (1984), applying the conceptual framework of adaptation to nursing encourages and allows examination of the dynamic interface between person and environment. For the purposes of this project, a literature review exploring the concepts of coping, burnout, long-term care, and occupational stress was conducted. Little research had been done regarding RNs and certified nursing assistants who work with dementia patients in long-term care and experience burnout. Nevertheless, mental health staff represents one of the categories of health workers at highest risk of burnout (Thomsen, Soares, Nolan, Dallender, & Arnetz, 1999). Burnout is a critical issue for mental health care delivery as it can lead to the decreased effectiveness of the workforce and poorer treatment outcomes (Priebe et al., 2004).

Standards of Care

It is recommended to target assessment for dementia when a patient exhibits decline in independent living and safety associated with memory or cognition changes, signs of mild cognitive impairment, learning disabilities, and stroke or neurological condition, such as Parkinson's disease (Alzheimer's Association,

2012). Basic activities of living such as bathing, dressing, grooming, and toileting should be assessed (Alzheimer's Association, 2012).

Tools for Early Identification of Dementia

Cognition assessment tools that have been validated to use for assessing cognition function include the Mini-Cognition assessment tool, Mini-Mental State Examination (MMSE), Montreal Cognitive Assessment (MoCA), and General Practitioner Assessment of Cognition (GPCOG) (USPSTF, 2003). The Mini-Cognition tool takes approximately two to four minutes to administer. A score below three is suggestive of dementia and indicates the need for additional dementia screening (USPSTF, 2003). MMSE is one of the most widely used tests and has high specificity (USPSTF, 2003). This test takes eight minutes to administer. A score lower than 24 is suggestive of dementia or delirium (USPSTF, 2003). MoCA is the most comprehensive test and has high sensitivity. This test takes approximately 10 minutes to administer, and a score lower than 26 is suggestive of dementia or mild cognitive impairment (USPSTF, 2003).

Diagnosis

A diagnosis of dementia should be made only after a thoughtful assessment to exclude other causes. Assessment includes a detailed history taking, cognitive and mental state examination, physical examination, and a review of medications (Alzheimer's Association, 2012). There are no clear data to support or refute ordering routine laboratory studies such as a complete blood count, electrolytes, glucose, and renal and liver function tests. A diagnosis of dementia cannot be made solely based on the results of any of the cognitive assessment tools. It also requires that functional status correlate well with the results (USPSTF, 2003). Tables 1 and 2 present symptoms and criteria for diagnosing dementia. Table 3 outlines major points of delivering the diagnosis.

Table 1

Diagnosing Dementia Using DSM-IV Criteria

Dementia Symptoms
1. Memory impairment 2. At least one of the following: a. Aphasia—inability to use and understand language; b. Apraxia—inability to perform learned movement; c. Agnosia—inability to recognize objects; d. Disturbance in executive functioning; e. Cognitive deficits significantly interfering with work, social activities, or relationships; and f. Cognitive deficits not occurring exclusively during delirium.

Note. See American Psychiatric Association (2013).

Table 2

Additional Criteria for Determining Dementia Type 1

Dementia Type	Prevalence 2	Common Signs/Symptoms
Alzheimer's Disease	50%	Gradual onset with continuing decline; Social withdrawal; Paranoia; Anxiety not caused by identifiable medical, psychiatric, or neuralgic condition.
Vascular Dementia	About 25%	Focal neurological signs or laboratory evidence of cerebrovascular condition (white-matter changes on imaging [although many patients with Alzheimer's disease also have such changes]; In general, a more stepwise decline compared to a more gradual decline of patients with Alzheimer's.
Lewy bodies dementia	15%	History of fluctuating cognitive performance; Well-formed visual hallucinations (unrelated to dopaminergic therapy); History of parkinsonism emerging simultaneously with cognitive impairment; Parkinson's associated dementia is characterized by onset of Parkinson's disease symptoms before dementia onset.
Dementia due to other causes [3]	5%	Evidence from history, physical exam or laboratory findings of a specific medical condition causing cognitive deficits (head trauma, HIV disease, Parkinson's disease, Huntington's chorea, Pick's disease, Creutzfeldt-Jakob disease). [4,5]

Note. [1]Adapted from American Psychiatric Association (2013). [2]See Burns & Iliffe (2009). [3]Includes mixed-cause cases (vascular and Alzheimer's dementias). [4]There is no clear data to support or refute ordering routine laboratory studies such as complete blood count, electrolytes, glucose, and renal and liver function tests. [5]There is no evidence for routine use of genetic markers. False positives may occur and would be emotionally and financially devastating.

Table 3

Delivering a Diagnosis of Dementia

Key considerations	A. Explain the biology of the disease and what to expect; B. Maintain independence as much as possible; and C. Create a safe environment.
Talking points	A. "Memory changes are due to abnormal accumulation of proteins in the brain, which interferes with the essential functions of thinking processing. Basically, these proteins clog things up"; B. "Eventually, dementia will cause a worsening in your ability to handle regular tasks, such as shopping, finances, and taking medications. But we'll talk regularly, and we'll manage that"; C. "Dementia is not hereditary in most cases"; D. "Dementia is a progressive condition with no cure, but we have treatments for symptoms. And proper care and planning can greatly alleviate the burden of dementia"; and E. "It is important for you and your family to plan for the future, and it is especially important for you to make legal plans. The sooner legal planning starts, the more you may be able to participate. Legal planning includes advance directives."

Treatment and Care Plan

It is important to include family in the treatment plan and goals. The type of support the patient and family or caregiver need will evolve with the progression of the disease. Families should be educated that inevitable disease-related deficits will develop in memory, behavior, mood, and function (National Institute for Health and Clincial Excellence, 2011). Lifestyle modification and non-pharmacologic options, such as exercise and introducing pleasant activities daily, can improve mood and increase quality of life. Day treatment programs and occupational therapy programs also improve quality of life for dementia patients (Alzheimer's Association, 2012).

The treatment plan may include the use of medications. When educating patients and families, it is important to tell them that medications may be helpful in slowing the rate of decline in cognitive function in some patients (Sobow & Kloszewska, 2007). If the treatment plan includes using medications, functional and behavioral goals should be developed with the patient and family to help maintain the checkbook, maintain a prescribed medication schedule, and increase social interaction (Boudreau et al., 2011). A plan of care should be created to monitor the medication's safety and effectiveness. Medication should be continued only as long as the patient's global functioning and behavioral conditions remain at a level where the drug is considered having a worthwhile effect

(Diniz et al., 2009). Table 4 presents the goals of dementia treatment.

Table 4

Goals of Treatment for Dementia

Disease Stage	Treatment Goals
Mild cognitive impairment/ memory loss	• Maintain function, safety, and independence; • Reduce or cease medication that may be contributing to decreased cognition.
Early-stage dementia	• Maintain function and independence while preserving safety; • Reduce or cease medication that may be contributing to decreased cognition.
Mid-stage dementia	• Preserve safety, function, and independence; • Develop skills that support continued living at home and delay institutionalization;
Late-stage dementia	• Preserve safety, comfort, and dignity;
End-stage dementia	• Consider hospice referral.

Care Facilities for Alzheimer's Type Dementia Patients

Alzheimer's is a progressive cognitive decline of the thought processes and physical decline of functional ability to care for oneself. The physical and mental demands on the family may become too exacting and overwhelming (Russell, de Benedictis, & Saisan, 2014). The patient may require total assistance with physical tasks such as bathing, dressing, and toileting as well as greater overall supervision (Russell et al., 2014).

Assisted living facilities and nursing homes with locked units are two main types of facilities that care for Alzheimer's type dementia patients. Assisted living is an option for families who need assistance with some activities of daily living. Staff is available 24 hours a day, and some facilities provide minor help with medication as well (Russell et al., 2014). Nursing homes with special care units for Alzheimer's patients should provide assistance in both activities of daily living and a high level of medical care (Russell et al., 2014). A medical director oversees the care provided at nursing homes where skilled nursing professionals specializing in psychiatric dementia care provide 24-hour care for patients (Russell et al., 2014). Alzheimer's units should have policy and procedures for caring for dementia type patients. There should be dedicated staffing according to patient acuity (Russell at al., 2014). Activities should be patient specific and should be implemented daily according to the patients' needs. Training and education in Alzheimer's type units should be planned monthly.

Psychiatric-Mental Health Nurses' Roles and Responsibilities

Psychiatric unit nurses are RNs specializing in the institutional care of large hospitals and medical centers that have patients staying in the unit for a short-term evaluation or at intensive treatment centers or in long-term care units (Nurses for a Healthier Tomorrow, 2014).

Psychiatric nurses work with patients with various mental and behavioral conditions that require them to focus on patient interaction. Psychiatric nurses care for patients with illness or disease that has led them to temporary or long-term hospitalization or psychiatric Alzheimer's units (Nurses for a Healthier Tomorrow, 2014). Psychiatric unit nurses are assigned to provide direct care to their patients, including facilitating social and emotional needs, supervising medication scheduling, and evaluating patient progress. Psychiatric nurses provide the best possible care by collaborating with a variety of interdisciplinary professionals (Nurses for a Healthier Tomorrow, 2014). Registered nurses (RNs) are also responsible for educating the patient's family about the patient's conditions and creating a supportive environment for the patient in long-term care, which is very important.

Psychiatric nurses are responsible for maintaining a safe environment with monitoring devices and restraining techniques when necessary. They encourage social support by creating and encouraging patients to take advantage of opportunities, such as support groups and social activities, and by redirecting patients in a calm, therapeutic manner if needed. Psychiatric nurses are the backbone of the mental health patient care and community. They are responsible for the direct care of patients, facilitating recovery through social interaction and traditional medical treatments.

Definition of Terms

1. *Burnout*—a key aspect of the burnout syndrome is increased feelings of emotional exhaustion (Maslach et al., 1996). Burnout is also characterized by depersonalization (also referred to as "cynicism") and reduced personal accomplishment (Maslach, 1982). Workload encompasses physical and emotional demands as well as the type of work and skills required.

   Workplace stress is the physical and emotional outcomes of a disparity between demands of the job and the amount of control the individual has in meeting those demands (Lambert & Lambert, 2008). As McShane and Von Glinow (2005) stated, if stress is not managed, it leads to burnout. Job burnout is the process by which emotional exhaustion, cynicism, and reduced efficacy occur due to the cumulative result of stress. For example, staff turnover sick days and angry outbursts are associated with burnout. Workers may feel unhappy about themselves and dissatisfied with their accomplishments on the job. Employees' lack of influence on decisions that affect their job may cause burnout—for example, hours of work, assignments they receive, inability to control the amount of work that comes in, unclear job expectations, dysfunctional work dynamics, poor job fit, and high acuity of patients (Mayo Clinic, n.d.).

2. *Coping*—a vital part of any person's survival in today's fast-paced health care environment. Lazarus and Folkman (1984) noted that "coping serves two overriding functions: managing or altering the problem with the environment causing distress (problem-focused coping) and regulating the emotional response to the problem (emotion-focused coping)" (p. 179). Lazarus defined coping as "not a single act but a constellation of many acts and thoughts engendered by a complex set of demands that may stretch out over time" (1998, p. 207). The choice of coping option is determined by internal and external factors. Personal agenda (e.g., beliefs, values, experience) and resources (e.g., financial or social support) influence the outcome.

   Coping behaviors are generally classified as problem-oriented strategies and affective-oriented (short-term) methods. The problem-oriented strategies are those used to solve stress-producing problems, whereas the affective-oriented methods manage the emotional component involved. Short-term coping methods (eating, sleeping, and smoking) help release professionals' feeling that their actions are not producing positive results (Maslach,

1982). Such short-term methods reduce tension temporarily but do not deal directly with the stressful situation. Drawing on past experiences and talking it out with others are examples of long-term stress-reduction methods as well. The problem-oriented strategies, however, are seen as constructive ways of dealing with stress (Keller, 1990).

3. *Mindfulness*—the state of being aware, present, attentive, and in the moment. Mindfulness is a non-judgmental way of being. The state of mindfulness can be attained through education, mentoring, or practice.

Conceptual and Operational Definition of Terms

1. *Stress*—conceptually defined as the physical, chemical, and emotional process that produces tension and can cause illness. Stress can be perceived as either positive or negative, although stress is generally considered negative. According to Maslach and Jackson (1981), there are many events that can cause negative stress for some individuals and positive stress for others. In other words, not all individuals are stressed by the same situation. Operationally, stress will be defined by responses to the DCL stress scale (Fagin et al., 1996) that will be used in this study to measure perceptions of stress. This instrument is a 30-item questionnaire. The DCL stress scale assesses responses related to activities experienced at work by the psychiatric nurse such as dealing

with disturbed and unpredictable patients, having a lack of promotion prospects, having to deal with colleagues who do not do their share of the work, and having too little time to plan and evaluate treatment.

2. *Coping*—a unique set of cognitions and behaviors that are activated by alarming events or excessive demands (stressors). The type of coping strategy utilized by individuals varies and is determined by a variety of factors. Operationally, coping will be defined by responses to the PsychNurse Methods of Coping Questionnaire (PNMCQ) (McElfatrick et al., 2000) that will be used in this study to measure the degree to which mental health nurses to deal with work-related stress utilize various coping strategies. Some of the items on the survey include the following: "I deal with stress by believing in and feeling good about myself"; "I deal with stress by managing my time efficiently"; and "I deal with stress by venting to a friend or loved one."
3. *Burnout*—a physical, mental, and emotional response to constant high levels of stress and ineffective or inadequate coping methods. Burnout produces a variety of feelings and behaviors including hopelessness, powerlessness, cynicism, resentment, stagnation, and reduced productivity. Operational definition of burnout will be provided by

responses to the MBI-Human Services Survey (MBI-HSS) (Maslach & Jackson, 1981) that will be utilized in this study to measure the frequency of burnout. The MBI-HSS consists of 22 statements asking the respondent to rate his or her feelings regarding a variety of situations. An example of the statements is "Professionals feel that their actions are not producing positive results" (Maslach, 1982).

Clinical Practice of Nurses and Burnout

The Work Environment

An estimated 500,000 RNs in the United States are not in the profession due to the difficult working conditions, limited staffing, and long hours (Herbst, 2007). Nurses make life-and-death decisions that may result in moral distress and ethical stress, which can lead to significant health consequences. A study found that 15% of nurses reported leaving their positions because of moral distress in the workplace (Corley, Elswick, Gorman, & Clor, 2001). Nurses now care for more patients during a shift, which has led to a number of problems for both nurses and patients. Understaffing contributed to nearly a quarter of the unanticipated problems that result in death or injury to hospital patients (Joint Commision on Accreditation of Healthcare Organizations, 2002).

According to the U.S. Bureau of Labor Statistics, U.S. Department of Labor (n.d.), overexertion resulted in 39% of RN injuries. Nurses' cardiovascular health suffers from working long shifts and overtime. In their study, Virtanen et al. (2010) showed a clear link between frequent overtime work and incidents of heart disease in nurses; workers who reported three to four hours of overtime work per day were 1.6 times more likely to have cardiovascular health disorders.

Many RNs complain that current workloads are causing burnout. A number of symptoms including irritability, insomnia, headache, back pain, weight gain, depression, and high blood pressure (Malugani, 2009) manifests chronic fatigue. Forty-nine percent of RNs under 30 and over 40 experienced high levels of burnout (Grove & Erickson, 2006). A study by Aiken, Clarke, & Sloane (2002) showed that when a registered nurse has over four patients, the risk of death for hospital patients increases by 7%.

While the American economy declined in 2009, the U.S. Bureau of Labor Statistics, U.S. Department of Labor (n.d.) projected nursing to become the number one profession in terms of growth. The increase in growth is largely due to the high turnover, vacancy rates, rising number of retiring baby-boomer generation nurses, and increased health care needs of patients. The current national vacancy rate in registered nursing is 8.1% and the demand continues to grow by about 2% each year (AACN, 2014). These rates are staggering to the American public and are considered a health care crisis for quality and safety of patient care (*Cost of Poor Quality*, 2008).

Nurses and Burnout

The most common source of stress and burnout among nurses is work overload brought on by inadequate staffing (Joint Commission, 2012). Studies, in which the Maslach Burnout Inventory (MBI) has been used, have shown that inadequate staffing correlates with a high score on the Emotional Exhaustion subscale (Aiken et al., 2002; GAO, 2001; Vahey et al., 2004). Increased workload is related to other factors besides actual patient volume, including extended shifts, overtime (often mandatory), many consecutive days of work, rotating shifts, weekend work, and on-call requirements. Increased levels of patient needs also contribute to work overload. A high level of care with short stays, unbalanced workload across various levels of care within the patient population, and nursing shortage are sources of burnout in nursing staff (Maslach, 2003; Vahey et al., 2004). The ongoing shortage is directly related to the high turnover among nurses because of burnout. Job dissatisfaction leads to burnout, nursing turnover, and inadequate staffing, which further increases job dissatisfaction (ANA, 2010). The nursing shortage is projected to grow more than 250,000 by 2025 (Buerhaus, Auerbach, & Staiger, 2009), which will increase burnout in the working population of nurses.

Further, research studies discuss significant stress nurses experience when caring for patients in hospital settings (Cronqvist, Theorell, Burns, & Lützén, 2001). The actual work of caring and attending to patient and family needs may create joy while at the same time subjecting nurses to work stress. Patient care can be complex and demanding. According to Shimizu, Mizoue, Kubota, Mishima, and Nagata (2003), nurses are at considerable risk for work-related stress. Caring for certain, types of patients such as those in chronic pain, psychiatric patients, and patients who are dying can be difficult and challenging. Nurses who work in these areas are at high risk for burnout. If stress is not managed effectively, it can lead to job dissatisfaction and potential health problems for nurses.

Patient Outcomes

Several studies have shown that decreased staffing, which results from burnout, poses a serious threat to patient safety and outcomes (Aiken et al., 2002; Kane, Shamliyan, Mueller, Duval, & Wilt, 2007; Stone, Du, & Gershon, 2007). Thus, ineffective communication between nurses and physicians significantly decreases the quality of patient care and causes increase in medication errors and inappropriate diagnosis and treatment of patients. Therefore, administration should offer training programs that focus on effective communication between nurses and physicians and on allowing health care professionals to interact outside of the patient's bedside (Rosenstein & O'Daniel, 2008; Smith, 2004). Interdisciplinary rounds, patient care seminars, continuing education lectures, and hospital committees can provide opportunities for nurses and physicians to collaborate on projects and gain a better understanding and respect for each other (Puntillo & McAdam, 2006; Smith, 2004).

CHAPTER II

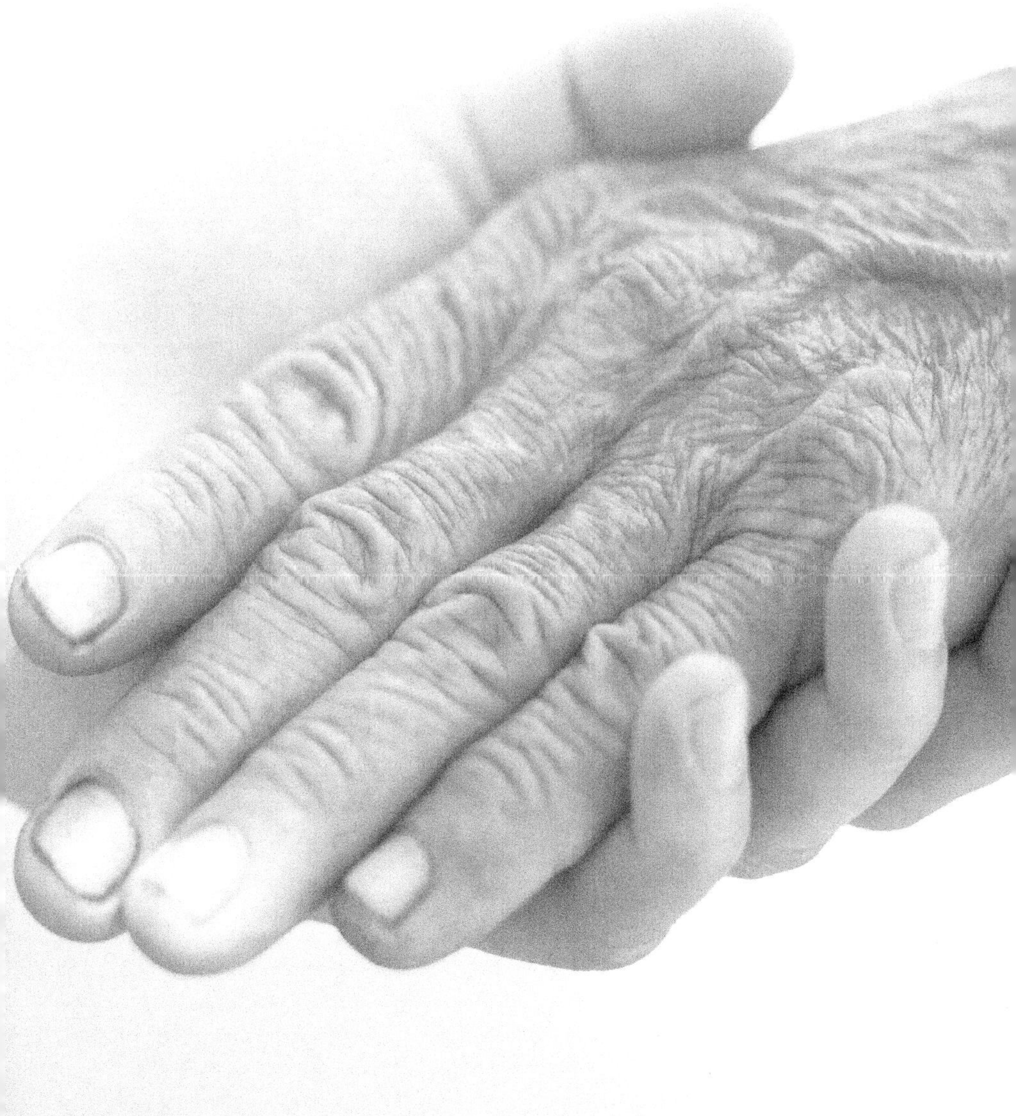

LITERATURE REVIEW

The objective of the literature review was to examine the existing body of knowledge pertaining to stress, coping, and burnout experienced by psychiatric nurses. The literature review provided a greater understanding of the concepts and occupation as well as guidance and organization for the ideas and theories relating to stress, coping, and burnout, especially in psychiatric units.

The researcher conducted a search of several databases including MEDLINE, CINAHL, World Wide Web Internet's Google Search Engine, ProQuest, PubMed, PubMed Central, PsychoINFO, and PsycARTICLES. For additional data, the researcher reviewed the following sources: Journal of Psychiatric and Mental Health Nursing, Journal of Advanced Nursing, International Journal of Nursing Studies, Journal of Psychological Nursing and Mental Health Services, and Journal of Clinical Nursing and Mental Health Nursing. The reviewed research studies focused on psychiatric nurses working in a variety of settings such as community mental health, forensic, and long-term facilities and hospitals. Studies were conducted all over the world with fifteen of the studies conducted in the United Kingdom, two in the United States, two in Australia, one in Sweden, and one in the Netherlands.

Psychiatric-Mental Health Nurses and Burnout

Three of the studies examined for the purposes of this project investigated occupational stress pertaining specifically to nurses working in acute mental health units. Thus, Jenkins and Elliott

(2004) set out to examine the relationship between stress and burnout among qualified and unqualified nursing staff (*N* = 93) working in acute adult mental health wards in the United Kingdom. Two groups of participants differed in their perceptions of stress. The main stressor for qualified staff was a lack of adequate staffing. The main stressor for unqualified staff was dealing with physically threatening, difficult, or demanding patients. Fifty percent of both groups demonstrated high levels of burnout. Other stressors reported by both groups included workload, client-related difficulties, organizational issues, conflicts with other professionals, lack of resources, professional self-doubt, and home-work conflict. These findings were consistent with the belief that job-related stressors lead to staff burnout.

In another study, Sullivan (1993) researched stressors identified by nursing staff (*N* = 61) working in the acute psychiatric in-patient facilities of two health authorities in the United Kingdom. The author also sought to assess the effects of stress and identify the types of coping strategies utilized by the nurses working in this setting. The results indicated that nurses most often cited the following stressors: violent incidents, potential suicides, and observation of patients. Other stressors reported included staffing levels, administrative duties, and feeling overworked. The most frequently utilized coping strategies were social support, problem solving, and avoidance techniques. Consistent with the results of previous studies, a high level of burnout was discovered in a majority of the nurses. Most importantly, reliability and validity were not reported in the study.

Further, a study conducted by Muscroft and Hicks (1998) in Birmingham, England, involved 50 psychiatric nurses and 50 general nurses in order to investigate occupational stress and coping of the two diverse groups of nurses. This study used questionnaires as a means of data collection. The results suggested the general nurses reported more occupational stress than psychiatric nurses did. It is important to note that the sample size of each group was relatively small.

Trygstad (1986) conducted a US-based study that consisted of semi-structured interviews with a sample of only 22 qualified nurses working in acute in-patient settings. The researcher was to identify work-related stressors and factors that assisted the nurses in coping. The results of this study indicated that the most important determinants of work-related stress reported were difficulties in nurses' relationships with either other RNs or the head nurse and the ability to work together. Unit staff relationships accounted for one third of all stressors identified; this included inadequate communication and fighting between individuals and groups in the unit. The sample size was extremely small ($N = 22$). Moreover, the study failed to specify whether the sample consisted of RNs, licensed practical nurses, or unlicensed staff.

Stress, Coping, and Burnout of Psychiatric Nurses Working in a Variety of Settings

Kilfedder et al. (2001) conducted a study that examined burnout among psychiatric nurses working in the United Kingdom. Subjects were psychiatric nurses ($N = 510$) employed in a Scottish Health Service Trust, which included a range of acute hospital and community settings. Several instruments were used to measure stress, coping, burnout, and job satisfaction. The psychiatric nurses in this study had lower levels of burnout compared to the normative data.

Next, Jeanneau and Armelius (2000) conducted a Sweden-based study about self-image and burnout among psychiatric staff. The sample consisted of mental health workers ($N = 754$) employed in a variety of mental health care settings including psychiatric wards, small psychiatric treatment homes, forensic wards, and community care centers. The researchers discovered that highly burned-out individuals had a significantly more negative self-image than staff who had rated themselves as experiencing low levels of burnout.

Finally, Melchior et al. (1996) conducted a study that examined the effectiveness of primary nursing interventions in decreasing burnout levels among psychiatric nurses in long-stay settings. A random sample of 161 psychiatric nurses from five psychiatric hospitals located in the Netherlands participated in this longitudinal study. The results indicated neither decrease nor increase in burnout levels after the primary nursing interventions had been introduced to the participants.

Stress, Coping and Burnout in Psychiatric Nursing Students

One study (Tully, 2004) reviewed for the purposes of this research examined stress and coping methods among psychiatric nursing students in the United Kingdom. Students (N = 35) were given a questionnaire in their 74th week of training. The author of the study discovered that students preparing to become nurses in a psychiatric setting were significantly stressed emotionally and that most of the stressors were specific to their education—the amount of information they were required to learn, exams, and fear of failure were most stressful. The students reported that they utilized coping methods such as comfort eating, drinking, smoking, taking medications, taking it out on others, and simply wishing things were different. The students reporting lower stress levels used more effective coping strategies such as talking to others, seeking advice, getting assistance, changing things so that the situation might improve, and taking things one step at a time.

Further, Kipping (2000) examined the experiences of stress among 440 psychiatric nursing students during their time as students and shortly after they began working as nurses in the United Kingdom. Major stressors for students included exams, assessments, written work, and placement and student issues. Once the students began their careers as psychiatric nurses, open-ended questions were utilized in order to provide details about the nature of stress. The nurses reported several aspects of their jobs as stressful including patient issues, coworker relationships, performance of other staff, changes, and administrative issues. The results of this study provide valuable information for nursing education and can be applied broadly to psychiatric nursing.

Stress, Coping, and Burnout in Community Health Nurses

Community mental health nurses work in the community rather than in hospitals or long-term care facilities. A study conducted by Pinikahana and Happell (2004) measured stressors and burnout levels and job satisfaction in community health nurses (N = 136) employed in rural mental health services in Victoria, Australia. The results of this study indicated that workload and inadequate preparation were reported most often as the most stressful situations. The majority of community health nurses were found to be satisfied with their jobs and only a fraction of the nurses were experiencing high levels of burnout. The exact type of work setting was not described in detail, and it is only known that the nurses in this study worked in rural and remote settings throughout Australia.

Stress, coping, and burnout among community health nurses were also the focus of the four separate studies conducted by Burnard, Edwards, Fothergill, Hannigan, & Coyle (2000); Edwards,

Burnard, Coyle, Fothergill, & Hannigan (2000, 2001); and Hannigan, Edwards, Coyle, Fothergill, & Burnard (2000). The researchers used questionnaires to explore stress, coping, and burnout among community health nurses (*N* = 301). The results indicated that community health nurses were experiencing high levels of stress and burnout. Half of the participants were found to be emotionally overextended and exhausted and therefore unable to provide quality care to their clients. The level of exhaustion was greater in community health nurses working in urban areas than in community health nurses working in rural areas. The most stressful aspects perceived by psychiatric community health nurses in these four studies were workload, poor resources, excessive paperwork, and management problems as well as a broad spectrum of client-related issues. Coping strategies utilized most often by the community health nurses included peer support, supervision, good communication skills, and a broad range of personal approaches, such as relaxation and confidence in one's own abilities.

Further, Snelgrove (1998) conducted a study on stress and job satisfaction in three diverse groups of nurses working in the United Kingdom. The sample groups included health visitors (*N* = 68), district nurses (*N* = 56), and CPNs (*N* = 19). Health visitors are nursing assistants who work in hospitals. District nurses are highly qualified nurses who have undergone further training to enable them to specialize in providing high-quality care to patients in the community. CPNs work specifically with psychiatric patients living either at home or in community-based treatment homes. All three groups of nurses as stressors reported organizational issues, lack of resources, and administrative issues. The results of the study indicated differences in the stress levels for each occupational group. Thus, health visitors reported the highest stress scores and lowest job satisfaction scores. District nurses had medium stress scores and low job satisfaction scores. CPNs also had medium stress scores and low job satisfaction scores. This study highlighted the importance of treating nurses according to their specialties rather than as a homogenous profession.

Fagin, Brown, Bartlett, Leary, & Carson (1995) conducted a comparison study to examine the stress levels of 250 CPNs and 323 ward-based psychiatric nurses in the United Kingdom. The study revealed comparisons between hospital-based psychiatric nurses and their community-based counterparts. A large proportion of both groups of nurses experienced high levels of stress and emotional exhaustion due to the demands of their work. The nurses who experienced high levels of stress used more sick time, experienced lower self-esteem, and felt unfulfilled in their work. Additionally, ward-based psychiatric nurses experienced greater feelings of depersonalization, or detachment from their patients, and a decreased sense of personal accomplishment in their work as compared to their colleagues working in the community (Fagin et al., 1995).

Research in Using Mindfulness-Based Stress Reduction by Health Professionals

Implementing programs to decrease job burnout and stress is needed for the nursing profession for the overall health and long tenure of nurses. Learning about self-care is a powerful health promotion for RNs who care for dementia-type patients in psychiatric units. Thus, Baker (2003) stated that increasing awareness and promoting a balanced life would improve the long-term survival of the health care professional. The mindfulness-based stress reduction (MBSR) program teaches mindfulness and loving-kindness towards self and others. Kabat-Zinn, Lipworth, and Burney (1985) designed an eight-week MBSR program. Participants attend a group for 2.5 hours per week and learn meditation, Hatha Yoga, and other formal and informal techniques to increase mindfulness. Supporting oneself with loving-kindness is the core of the program and the first step to the mindfulness activities in this course. The MBSR program consists of progressive mindfulness exercises to create awareness and openness in the individual. MBSR may be described as naturalistic and non-deliberate (Grossman, Niemann, Schmidt, & Walach, 2004).

Although several MBSR studies focusing on health professions have been conducted, neither study has focused on RNs alone. The next section of this chapter discusses the research findings on the use of MBSR by health professionals.

Quantitative Studies of Using MBSR by Health Professionals

Cohen-Katz et al. (2005) implemented a randomized control design study using the MBSR program as an intervention. The purpose of this study was to examine whether the MBSR program would decrease burnout and psychological distress and increase mindfulness in hospital staff. The Maslach Burnout Inventory (MBI), Brief Symptom Inventory (BSI), and the Mindfulness Attention Awareness Scale (MAAS) were used as psychometric instruments. The inclusion criteria for this study was regular contact with patients, employment at the hospital, being English speaking, and being over 18 years of age. Staff members with substance abuse problems or active tendencies of suicide were excluded from this study. Consent was obtained from 27 staff; 14 were randomized to the intervention group, and 13 were put in the wait-list group. Ninety percent of the staff members were nurses and the others were in supportive roles such as pastoral care, respiratory therapy, and social work. Time to attend the MBSR program and its cost were paid by the administration and the wellness program.

Measurement tools were administered prior to the intervention, immediately afterwards, and three months post-intervention. In this study, there was a 7% attrition rate in the intervention group. The mean age of the nursing staff was 46; 100% of the participants were female.

No significant differences were found between the intervention group and the wait-list group prior to the intervention aimed at increasing mindfulness and decreasing burnout and psychological distress. However, statistically significant positive differences occurred between the intervention group and the wait-list group on the mean scores post-intervention for mindfulness. Post-intervention scores on the MBI scale indicated a significant difference. A significant difference was also found for personal accomplishment in the intervention group immediately post-intervention but not at the three-month point.

A within-group analysis of the intervention group demonstrated significant reduction in emotional exhaustion on the MBI scale immediately post-intervention and three months later. The number of nurses with psychological distress recorded before the intervention decreased in both the intervention group and the wait-list group but not significantly.

Randomized control design and gaining the knowledge of the use of MBSR by health professionals in acute care settings were the strengths of this study. The limitations of the study included the small sample size, homogeneity of the sample, and bias introduced by paying the MBSR program course fees for the hospital staff.

Further, in their study, Galantino, Baime, Maguire, Szapary, and Farrar (2005) evaluated the relationship between physical and psychological stress measures before and after MBSR. Eighty-four health care employees participated in a quantitative nonrandomized research study on using the MBSR program. The health care employees participating in the study included managers and direct care givers from a university hospital setting. Ninety-six percent of the participants were female with a mean age of 43. Stress was measured by salivary cortisol levels collected between 5 p.m. and 7 p.m. The Profile of Mood States-Short Form (POMS-SF) was used to evaluate levels of stress and mood disturbances; MBI was used to evaluate burnout; and the Interpersonal Reactivity Index (IRI) was used to evaluate empathy.

Eighty-two percent of the participants completed all of the questionnaires, and 61% completed the pre- and post-cortisol test. No significant findings were reported for the cortisol levels from baseline. Statistically significant findings occurred from baseline in the Emotional Exhaustion subscale of MBI and the subscales of the POMS-SF scale. There were no changes in salivary cortisol over time; this study did not demonstrate a correlation between the cortisol level and the various psychological measures.

The strengths of this study included adequate sample size and gaining further knowledge of the outcomes of using the MBSR program. Patient satisfaction improved a quarter after MBSR was implemented, which may suggest long-term effects. The limitations of this study were lack of a control group, nonrandomized design, and the significant attrition. It was also unclear from the description of the sample whether the managers were clinically prepared and in what clinical area the health care professionals specialized.

Next, Mackenzie et al. (2006) conducted a study using a sample of 30 nurses and nursing assistants. It was a randomized control pilot study of the efficacy of a condensed version of MBSR utilizing the two works and experience of Kabat-Zinn (1990) and Segal, Willams, and Teasdale (2002) to compare a wait-list group and a control, or intervention, group. The intervention group had four 30-minute group sessions. Research subjects were instructed to practice 10 minutes per day, five days per week compared to 45 minutes per day, six days per week in the traditional MBSR program developed by Kabat-Zinn (1990).

Psychological measures were completed at baseline and post-training. MBI, the Smith Relaxation Dispositions Inventory (SRDI), Intrinsic Job Satisfaction subscale of the Job Satisfaction Scale (JSS), Satisfaction with Life Scale (SWLS), and Antonovsky's Orientation to Life Questionnaire were used to measure overall well-being. Repeated measures of analysis of variance (ANOVA) were performed on the effects of group participation over time on the subscales of burnout, sense of coherence, life satisfaction, relaxation, and work satisfaction.

Statistically significant effects were found in emotional exhaustion, depersonalization, and job-related personal accomplishments between the intervention group and the wait-list group. Participants who had completed the mindfulness program expressed significant satisfaction with life, well-being, and relaxation ratings. No significant findings were obtained for work satisfaction or sense of coherence.

The strengths of this study were the randomized control design and added knowledge of the effect of MBSR in nurses and nursing assistants. The methodological section was well written and clearly outlined the psychometric tools and their reliability. The limitations of this study included small sample size and heterogeneity of the sample, which consisted of two types of health professionals. It was unclear if the researchers controlled for outside factors that might have influenced the psychological parameters. This was the only study found during the literature review that modified the MBSR program and examined efficacy in a clinical setting.

Schenström, Rönnberg, and Bodlund (2006) conducted a prospective pilot study focusing on 52 health professionals in a primary care setting in Sweden. The purpose of this study was to explore the feasibility and usefulness of mindfulness and cognitive attitude training for health care professionals as well as to examine psychological factors related to well-being. The sample consisted mostly of physicians ($N = 29$), other health care professionals ($N = 23$) included nurses, physical therapists, occupational therapists, and social workers. Two physicians taught 50 hours of didactic and cognitive attitude exercises and mindfulness based on the MBSR program over a course of several weeks. MASS, the WHO-5 Well-Being Index, and two visual analog scales to measure stress were utilized pre-intervention, immediately post-intervention, and three months post-intervention. A questionnaire was provided to assess the intensity of mindfulness training at home.

Statistically significant increases in mindfulness and well-being occurred after the completion of the MBSR program. Reductions in stress were significant and were also reported on both visual analog scales. Those participants who practiced mindfulness more frequently reported a statistically significant increase in mindfulness immediately post-intervention and at the three-month follow-up.

The strengths of this study included a low dropout rate and longitudinal focus achieved through measures at three months post-intervention. The limitations of this study included lack of a control group, no randomization, and the use of the untested MAAS tool on Swedish population. In addition, due to the combination of MBSR with cognitive attitude training, it is unclear which program created the significant improvement in well-being.

Finally, Shapiro et al. (2005) conducted a prospective, randomized, controlled pilot study focusing on 38 participants employed in a health care setting. The sample included physicians, nurses, social workers, physical therapists, and psychologists randomized to either the MBSR intervention or a wait list. The purpose of the study was to examine the effects of MBSR on health care professionals currently working in clinical settings. Tools included BSI, the Perceived Stress Scale (PSS), SWLS, MBI, and the Self-Compassion Scale (SCS). Forty-four percent of the 18 participants in the intervention group and 10% of the 20 participants in the control group dropped out of the study. Statistically significant improvements in stress and self-compassion occurred in the intervention group. No statistically significant improvement in decreasing burnout rates was observed.

The strengths of this study included using the randomized control design and contributing to further knowledge of using MBSR by health professionals. High attrition rate and small sample size were limitations of the study. The intervention group may have had more of an improvement in stress due to the higher rate of stress at baseline than the control group. Selection bias may have occurred in both groups, as it is probable that those with higher amounts of stress or those for whom MBSR was not effective or palatable dropped out.

Qualitative Study of Using MBSR by Health Professionals

Cohen-Katz et al. (2005) conducted a qualitative design study on the same cohort they used for the quantitative arm of their study. Ninety percent of the 27 participants were nurses working in a variety of patient care units in the hospital. Reasons for participating in the study were family stress—aging, illness, or recent death of a family member. Three percent of the participants reported the stress of working part-time and performance anxiety at work. Twenty-seven percent reported demanding jobs, and 21% reported learning a new job as the main reason for work-related stress.

Qualitative data analysis included review of 46 open-ended questions given during the MBSR program, two interviews with the vice-president for patient care, and a one-hour focus group with seven of the 27 participants. Each of the researchers independently transcribed and reviewed the interviews recorded during the focus group. Content and themes were obtained from the transcripts, utilizing a 6-item codebook developed by the research team. Consensus was reached through two of the three researchers' agreeing on the coding for five test transcripts. The remaining documents were coded by the principal investigator and reviewed by the research team. The NVIVO software was used after the consensus coding. Themes that emerged from the focus-group interviews were "increase in empathy and appreciation of others," "increased relaxation," and "learning how to be in the present moment." Other themes were "patience," "calmness," "letting go of worry," and "being fully present in relationships."

The strengths of this study included using the grounded theory approach to analyzing themes, the explanation of the interpretative descriptions, and validation of the data through several coders and consensus, which increased reliability (Sandelowski & Barroso, 2003). The report is organized by section headers and includes the language of the participants. The singular focus group was a limitation of this study. It was unclear from the study description if long-term effects occurred. Finally, the research team should have mentioned if the participants validated the transcripts for accuracy.

Many hospitals are implementing techniques to improve the work environment and conditions, utilizing quality-improvement and efficiency methods to help remove barriers for the delivery of high quality of care. Personal control over difficult situations begins with identification of stressors and accepting the responsibility to manage stress (Miller & Smith, 1993). Reframing stress and burnout and viewing situations as a whole help to manage the situation. Self-care programs are needed in locked Alzheimer's type dementia units to guide nurses in their management of stress and development of inner self. Through teaching nurses to stabilize and maintain inner balance and prevent stress and burnout, these programs may lead to improvement in nursing practice, personal health of nurses, and overall retention of the nursing workforce.

The findings of the quantitative and qualitative studies discussed above are useful in guiding the development of intervention programs for psychiatric nurses to assist in increasing nurses' job satisfaction, decreasing stress and burnout, enhancing positive coping mechanisms, and improving the overall health and well-being of nurses. Mindfulness practices are rooted in the philosophical Buddhist teaching and practices in Tibetan culture (Kabat-Zinn, 1990). The MBSR program produces psychological and physical outcomes that benefit the participants' overall state of well-being. The MBSR program will be useful in everyday practice for psychiatric nurses working in locked units, for orientation programs for psychiatric RNs working in locked units, and for continuing education programs. This program aims to expand knowledge of mindfulness as it relates to potential benefits to nurses and their work performance and effectiveness, which will improve quality of care.

In summary, several reviewed studies have shown promising outcomes in nursing staff currently working in health care. The studies that focused on nurses and nursing assistants working in hospital settings demonstrated a statically significant increase in mindfulness and significant decrease in emotional exhaustion (Cohen-Katz et al., 2005; Mackenzie et al., 2006).

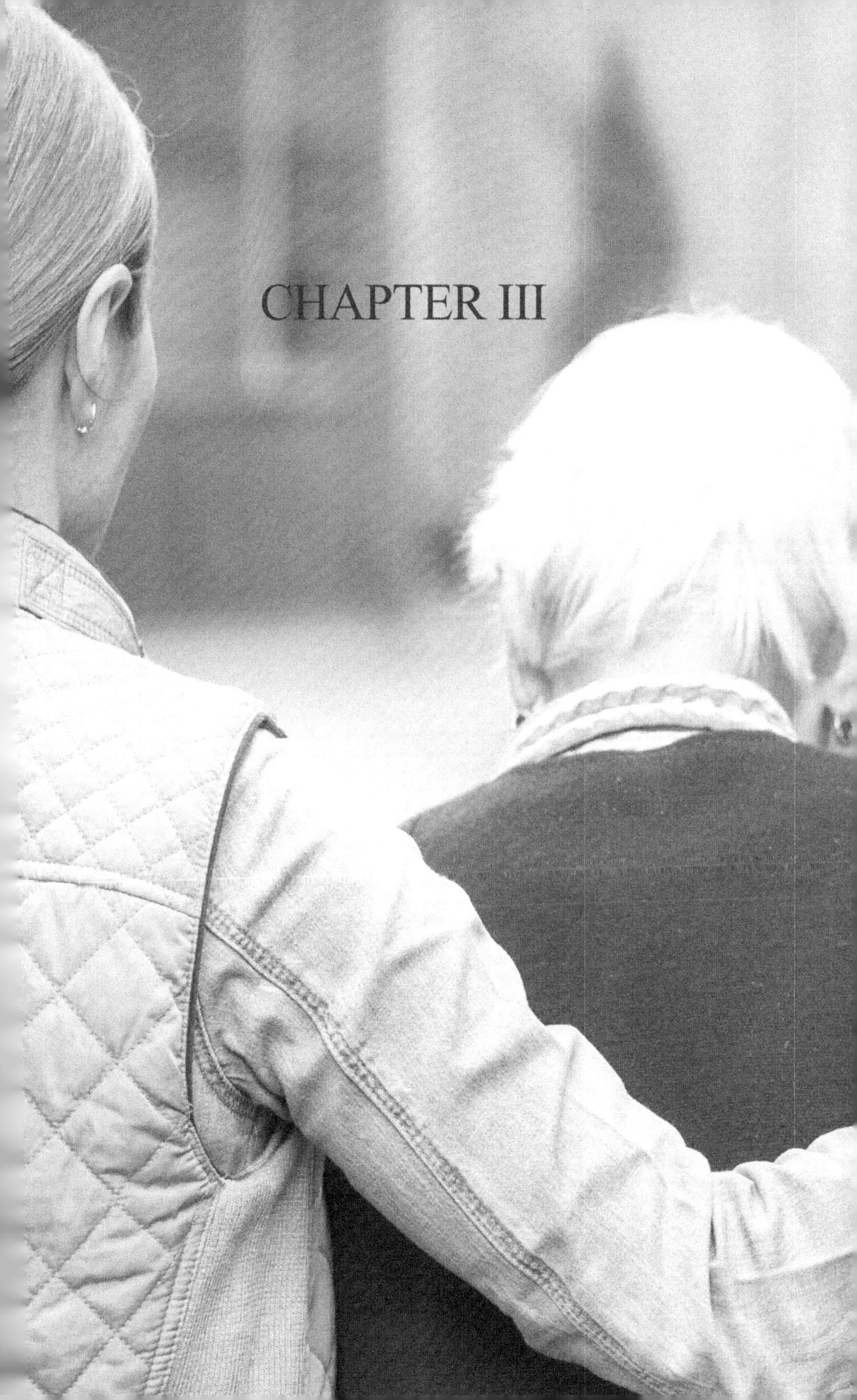

CHAPTER III

METHODOLOGY

Conceptual Framework

The conceptual framework of this project consists of several theoretical works conducted by three well-established theorists. A conceptual framework is a set of coherent ideas or concepts organized in a way that makes them easy to communicate to others. The purpose of this project is to decrease the perception of occupational stress and burnout in psychiatric-mental health nurses who provide direct care in psychiatric units to Alzheimer's type dementia patients. In the process of the project, the burnout and occupational stressors perceived by psychiatric nurses will be measured. The implementation of an MBSR intervention should reduce the perception of stress, will be measured by giving pre-, and post-tests of the previous MBI-HSS scale in a post-one-month period after MBSR has been implemented. In order to approach this task in an organized and scientific manner, three theoretical models will be used as a guide: Selye's (1974) stress health promotion theory, Lazarus and Folkman's (1984) coping theory, and Dorothea Orem's self-care theory (Taylor, 2006).

Theoretical Framework

Nursing Theories

The following major assumptions of Dorothea Orem's self-care theory are the basis of this MBSR program: (1) people should be self-reliant and responsible for their own care and others in family needing care, (2) nursing is a form of action between two or more persons, and (3) a person's knowledge of potential health problems is necessary for promoting self-care behaviors (Tomey & Alligood, 2002). According to Orem's theory, the goal of nursing is to render the patient or members of his or her family capable of meeting the patient's self-care needs. However, nurses must maintain a normal state of health and be balanced in order to care for others (Taylor, 2006). Dorothea Orem's general theory of nursing consists of three parts: theory of self-care, theory of self-care deficit, and theory of nursing systems (Taylor, 2006).

Dorothea Orem's universal self-care requisites include life processes and the maintenance of the integrity of human structure and functioning; balance between activity and rest and between solitude and social interaction; and prevention of hazards to human life, well-being, and promotion of human functioning (McEwen & Wills, 2002). This theory directs clinical practice for a supportive, educative system to improve nurses' health and the quality of care for this population.

Dorothea Orem's theory provides a comprehensive base for nursing practice. It has utility for professional nursing in the areas of nursing practice, nursing education administration, and nursing research. Dorothea Orem's theory is a contemporary approach—specific to nursing—with the concepts of health promotion and health maintenance.

Stress

Hans Selye, a Canadian endocrinologist and renowned stress theorist, defined stress as "the nonspecific responses of the body to any demand made upon it" (Selye, 1974, p. 27). He called it the general adaptation syndrome (GAS). GAS has three distinguishable phases: alarm, resistance, and exhaustion. These three phases occur sequentially. When stress sounds the alarm, initiates GAS, and is not removed or coped with, the body progresses into resistance and eventual exhaustion. Recovery is an outcome alternative to exhaustion when the source of stress is either removed or coped with effectively (Selye, 1956). Selye believed that the effects of the resistance phase of GAS result in the gradual wearing down of what he characterized as "weak link"—body parts or systems. This causes the body to be overwhelmed with stress and exhaustion.

Coping

Richard Lazarus is another well-accepted stress theorist. Lazarus developed a unique model explaining how our minds work when perceiving potential stressors. Lazarus' theory of psychological stress revolves around the belief that people or things become stressed when they feel something threat their well-being in some way. The threat can be either psychological or physiological in nature, and the perception of the stimuli determines whether they become stressors (Lazarus, 1966). Lazarus called the perception of potential stressors "threat" and the actual evaluation of stimuli threat, which is stress, "the appraisal process." Primary appraisal determines whether the stressor is a threat; the second appraisal determines whether the individual is capable of coping with the threat; and the third appraisal—the cognitive reappraisal—draws on the information from the first two appraisals (Lazarus & Lazarus, 1996).

According to Lazarus and Folkman (1984), stress is a real or perceived imbalance between the environment and an individual's ability to cope with or adapt to the imbalance. Individuals endure by continually coping with or adapting to the demands of a constantly changing environment.

Conceptual Links of Theory

Dorothea Orem believed nurses must maintain a normal state of health and be balanced in order to care for others. Dr. Syle believed that the usefulness of transcendental meditation technique prepares the nervous system to relax so that it can live with stress better. Lazarus Folkman (1984) believed individuals endure by continuously coping with or adapting to the demands of a constantly changing environment. These three theorists believed in a stress response and the body must find a positive way to cope in order to be balanced and healthy in everyday life processes. These theorist help support the concept of implementing the mindfulness based stress reduction intervention program to decrease the perception of stress and burnout in psychiatric nurses who work on locked units.

Aims of the Program

The aim of this program is to determine whether an MBSR intervention will decrease the perception of stress and burnout in nurses who work in Alzheimer's type dementia psychiatric units. The idea for implementing the program originated with the researcher's desire to improve the psychological well-being of registered nurses (RNs) working as staff nurses as well as the nursing care given by these nurses to patients with Alzheimer's type dementia.

Program Design and Setting

The quantitative program design targets RNs working in an Alzheimer's type dementia locked unit in a rural southern Mississippi hospital setting. The primary goal of implementing this program is to test the effectiveness of an MBSR intervention and to analyze whether the perception of stress and burnout will decrease post-intervention in RNs who care for patients with Alzheimer's type dementia. Standardized measures of the Maslach Burnout

Inventory–Human Services Survey (MBI–HSS) will be given pre- and post-MBSR intervention.

Program Participants

The target population for this program is psychiatric RNs working in a locked psychiatric unit within a small rural hospital in southern Mississippi. Each participant has to be (a) male or female, (b) 18 years of age or older, (c) employed either part- or full-time, (d) currently working in a locked psychiatric unit, (e) a Mississippi resident, and (f) currently licensed as an RN in Mississippi. Exclusion criteria required that participants be under the age 18 years, licensed practical nurses, nursing assistants, and nurse managers.

Methods of Measurement

The Maslach Burnout Inventory-Human Services Survey (MBI-HSS)

The Maslach Burnout Inventory–Human Services Survey (MBI-HSS) is a 22-item self-report measure of burnout (Maslach et al., 1996). MBI-HSS is used for workers that spend time with other people. The items are grouped into three subscales: Emotional Exhaustion, Depersonalization, and Personal Accomplishment. Emotional Exhaustion subscale is characterized by items such as "I am emotionally drained from my work." Depersonalization captures negative attitudes towards patients with items such as "I feel I treat some recipients as if they were impersonal objects." Finally, Personal Accomplishment subscale assesses how the individual evaluates himself or herself, particularly in relation to working with clients. This subscale includes such items as "I have accomplished many worthwhile things in this job." Items are rated on Likert-type scales from 0 = *never* to 6 = *every day*. Higher scores on Emotional Exhaustion and Depersonalization subscales reflect higher levels of burnout, whereas low scores on Personal Accomplishment subscale indicate high levels of burnout.

In Maslach et al.'s (1996) sample, internal consistency reliability coefficients (Cronbach's alpha) for the subscales were .922 for Emotional Exhaustion, .616 for Depersonalization, and .742 for Personal Accomplishment, with Depersonalization falling below the conventional .70 adequacy range. Test-retest reliability assessed by other researchers has ranged from low to moderately high, and all reliability testing for this scale's coefficients was significant beyond the .001 level. The MBI-HSS has also been found to have moderate convergent and discriminant validity. The tool was originally designed to be used in human services including nursing services.

Assumptions

1. Perception of burnout can be measured.

2. MBSR programmatic interventions can decrease the perception of stress and burnout in nurses and improve patient outcomes.

PICOT Question

The following PICOT question will guide this project:

1. Will implementing a mindfulness-based stress reduction (MBSR) program decrease the perception of stress and burnout and improve coping mechanisms in psychiatric nurses who care for patients with Alzheimer's type dementia?

Program and the DNP Essentials

This program will implement an MBSR intervention to decrease the perception of stress and burnout and improve coping mechanisms. The American Association of the Colleges of Nursing (AACN) (2006) describes the eight Doctorate of Nursing Practice (DNP) essentials for evidence-based practice. Implementation of this project will meet seven of the eight DNP essentials as presented in Table 5.

Table 5

DNP Essentials and the Project's Compliance

DNP Essentials	Project's Compliance
I. Organizational and systems leadership for quality improvement and systems thinking	Implementing this program will decrease burnout in RNs and will improve staff morale as well as organizational systems while decreasing staff turnover and sick days.
II. Clinical scholarship and analytical methods for evidence-based practice	This program has opportunities to disseminate evidence-based practices based on best-practice findings. Leadership and advocacy will be implemented with the program.
III. Information system/technology and patient care technology for the improvement and transformation of health care	Information systems and technology will be used to evaluate and look up evidence-based practice regarding burnout. The program will be placed in organizational technology systems for educational purposes.
IV. Health care policy for advocacy in health care	The program can be implemented into policy of organization for new hires and used in ongoing training for burnout annually through staff development.
V. Interprofessional collaboration for improving patient and population health outcomes	This program can be presented to other facilities as a consultation program for RNs to decrease stress in locked psychiatric units.
VI. clinical prevention and population health for improving the nation's health	This program will involve risk reduction and will prevent or decrease burnout thus improving health care outcomes.
VII. Advanced nursing practice	This program can be utilized in advanced nursing practice to implement education and prevent burnout in nurses. It can be used as scientific underpinnings for practice by improving quality of care in this population.

Note. See AACN (2006).

The DNP's role is being patients' advocate and leader while addressing health care disparities in the community. The goal of the intervention is to decrease the perception of stress and burnout in RNs who care for Alzheimer's type dementia patients in locked psychiatric units and thus to improve nurse-patient interactions and patient outcomes.

Sources of data.

The data analysis will include descriptive analysis of the demographic tool.

Data analysis.

The data analysis will include analysis of the results of the Maslach Burnout Inventory-Human Services Survey (MBI-HSS).

Ethics and human subject issues.

After obtaining the University of Southern Mississippi's Institutional Review Board's (IRB) approval, the researcher will implement the project focusing on RNs working in a locked psychiatric unit in a rural area of southern Mississippi and caring for patients with Alzheimer's type dementia.

Program Implementation

MBI-HSS will be administered to the participants before implementing the MBSR program. The measurement scales will be re-administered two weeks later to reassess the participants' perception of stress and burnout coping behavior after the implementation of the program. The program will include four two-hour group sessions of mindfulness-based stress reduction. This program will be implemented four Saturdays at 45 minutes per session. Further, the participants will be asked to practice 5-15 minutes per day of informal practice, five days per week for four weeks. During program implementation, periodic breaks will be allowed so the participants can relax and informally discuss the ideas that have been presented. Visual aids will be used to allow the participants to see what they are hearing. The setting will be arranged in a less formal way for the participants to see each other and the presenter. This will allow for interaction between the study participants.

Upon the implementation of this program, the researcher will stay on schedule, call the participants by name, provide appropriated handouts, summarize ideas in periodic intervals, schedule breaks for the participants, ask open-ended questions, and start and finish on time. After the implementation of the program, the researcher will follow up with a question-and-answer session to assess if the participants are applying ideas learned during the MBSR program implementation.

Mindfulness-Based Stress Reduction Key Concepts Structure, Methods, and Program Objectives

Structure and Methods

A. Group Pre-Program Orientation (2.5 Hours) explaining program administering The Maslach Burnout Inventory-Human Services Survey (MBI-HSS) to access level of burnout before implementation of program. Informed consents will be signed for participation if needed. Objectives will be covered and a verbal presentation will be given on how mindfulness stress reduction can decrease stress and improve coping in their professional life and everyday life of nurses. Explain the profound impact of burnout syndrome on nursing.

B. Four-weekly classes every Saturday for (2 hours) in duration.

C. "Formal" Mindfulness Mediation Methods will be presented with group participation.

   a. Body scans Medication-sitting and supine in a chair medication focusing on concentrating on tight parts of your body, internally at that time without distractions. (15 minutes approximated time each session).

   b. Gentle Hatha Yoga-Practiced with mindfulness awareness of the body in calm quite environment. This contains light stretching exercises. For example, shoulder rolling, neck rolls, sitting in a chair, bending forward to touch toes, holding for 5 to 10 seconds, and returning to sitting position. (At no time will I touch the participants). 15 minutes approximated time each session.

c. Sitting Mediation-Mindfulness of breath, body, feelings, thoughts, emotions and choice less awareness. Breathing exercises will be implemented with cleansing breaths inhaling through nose and exhaling out through nose and exhaling out through the mouth. (15 minutes approximated time).

D. "Informal "Mindfulness Medication Practices (mindfulness in everyday life) will be taught. (Lecture 30 to 45 minutes with questions and answer sessions.

a. Awareness of pleasant and unpleasant events and your surroundings.

b. Awareness of breathing. Will illustrate cleansing breaths and how to refocus on task to decrease stress.

c. Deliberate awareness of routine activities and events such as eating, weather, driving, walking, and awareness of interpersonal communication with oneself.

E. Daily homework assignments will be given which consist of a minimum of 45 minutes per day of formal mindfulness practice and 5-15 minutes of informal practice, 6 days per week for the entire duration of the program.

a. It is expected for the participants to write down any exploration of hindrances of mindfulness and development and integration of mindfulness in daily task and at work. It is expected for the participants to communicate individually and participate in-group dialogue about their experiences. (Group participation deepens the experience and gives a therapeutic dialogue on an individual bases). CASE studies will be presented to the group to explore different situations to use mindfulness in personal life and professional life. EACH CLASS SESSION EVERY SATURDAY FOR FOUR WEEKS WILL PRACTICE FORMAL AND INFORMAL MINDDFULNESS AND DISCUSS HOMEWORK IN A GROUP SETTING.

F. Incorporation of the post assessment instrument the (MBI-HSS) to access level of burnout after program implementation.

a. Total in-class hours:30 hours
b. Total homework assignments: 36-40 hours
c. Total group Orientation Session time: 2.5 hours

Key Characteristics of Mindfulness Program:

1. A fundamental component to improve self-care
2. Training in mindfulness meditation
3. Educational orientation
4. Group format 10-40 participants
5. Individually tailored Instructions when needed
6. Highly participatory format with group
7. Strong support system
8. Self-responsibility within the context of a collaborative relationship between participant, and MBSR provider
9. Interactive dialogue between instructor and participate dialogue to explore perception, mental and behavioral habits and part tens that may inhibit learning, growth, healing and stress reduction.
10. Short-term intervention: This MBSR is a brief duration (4-weeks). The structure is intended to foster participant self-regulation and reliance.

Objectives:

1. Participants should be able to apply MBSR in their personal life and professional practice.
2. Participants should be able to practice three mindfulness meditation techniques.
3. Participants should recognize how stress is expressed in the body and mind. (BODY SCAN TECHIQUE).

4. Participants will use techniques to maintain and regain composure during a busy word day.
5. Understand the profound impact of burnout syndrome on nursing.

Potential Benefits

Potential benefits from participating in this project include improved coping mechanisms and decreased perception of stress and burnout in nursing staff caring for Alzheimer's type dementia patients in long-term care settings. This project will help the participants develop positive coping mechanisms and decrease the perception of stress and burnout. This intervention has the potential to improve nurses' productivity and quality of care. This project may also decrease staff turnover and improve retention.

Risks

Minimum risk is involved in the participation in this project. The researcher will educate the administrators and the director of nursing, who is an RN, on the subject of protecting human research participants. The researcher will make an oral presentation prior to obtaining informed consent for program participation to assure understanding of the program components. Participation is voluntary, and the researcher will obtain informed consent from all subjects before conducting the program to assure voluntary participation. All registered nurses (RNs) have the right to withdraw informed consent during any part of the program without penalty.

If the participants experience any emotional distress related to coping or burnout, a licensed advanced psychiatric practice nurse will be available. There is always a risk that questions on burnout pre- or post-test will make participants uncomfortable or anxious. Those who participate in this study will be reassured that this program is only intended to improve their level of knowledge and perception of the perception of burnout, stress, and coping.

Program Duration and Location

The proposed project will be presented in a locked psychiatric unit for patients with Alzheimer's type dementia on a locked unit located in rural southern Mississippi. The meeting room is spacious enough to comfortably accommodate the participating nursing staff and to provide sufficient room for privacy when answering questions. Approximately two hours will be allotted for the oral presentation and completion of informed consent forms, the scales, and demographic survey forms. One hour will be allotted for the evaluation of the program.

REFERENCES

American Association of Colleges of Nursing (AACN). (2006, October). *The essentials of doctoral education for advanced nursing practice.* Retrieved from http://www.aacn.nche.edu/publications/position/DNPEssentials.pdf

American Association of Colleges of Nursing (AACN. (2009, June 10). *American Association of Coleges of Nursing*. Retrieved from Nursing shortage fact sheet: http://aacn.nche.edu

AbuAlRub, R. (2004). Job stress, job performance, and social support among hospital nurses. *Journal of Nursing Scholarship*, 36(1), 73-78.

AHRQ. (2008, August 1). *Agency for Healthcare Research and Quality*. Retrieved from Hospital nurse staffing and quality of care: http://ww.ahrq.gov

Aiken LH, C. S. (2002). Hospital nurse staffing and patient mortality, nurse burnotu and job dissatisfaction. *JAMA*, 288(16): 1987-1993.

Aiken, L. C. (2002). Hospital nurse staffing and patient mortality, nurse burnout, and job dissatisfaction. *Journal of the American Medical Association*, 288(16),1987-1993.

Andrews, D. &. (2009). The Importance of Mental Health to the Experience of Strain: and Evidenced-guided approach to improve rentention. *Journal of Nursing Mangement*, 17(3), 340-351.

AP, S. (2004). Partners at the bedside: the importance of nurse-physician relationships. *Nurs Econ*, 22(3):161-164.

AP, S. (2004). Partners at the beside: the imprtance of nurse-physician relationships. *Nurse Economy*, 22(3):161-164.

Association, A. (2013). Alzheimer's disease facts and figures. *Alzheimers Dement*, 8(2):131-168.

Association, A. P. (2013). *Diagnostic and Statistical Manual of Mental Disorders: DSM-IV 6th ed.* Washington, DC.

Associaton., A. N. (2010, April). *Safe Nursing Staffing Poll Results.* Retrieved from http://www.safestaffingsaveslives.org/What isANADoing/PollResults.aspx.

azarus, R. &. (1984). *Stress, appraisal and coping.* New York: Springer.

Baba, V. V. (1999). Occupational mental health: A study of work - related depression among nurses in the Caribean. *International Journal of Nursing Studies*, 36, 163-169.

Baker, E. (2003). *Caring for ourselves: A therapists guide to personal and professional well-being.* Washington, DC: American Psychological Association.

Balevre, P. (2001). Professional nursing burnout and irrational thinking. *Journal for Nurses in Staff Development*, 17(5), 264-271.

Beeber, A. S. (2010). Challenges and Strategies for Implementing and Evaluating Dementia Care Staff Training in Long-Term Care Settings. *Alzheimer's Care Today*, 11:1,17-39.

Berling, J. (2001). Drowing not waving: Bunout and mental health nursing. *Contemporary Nurse*, 11(2-3), 247-259.

Boudreau DM, Y. O. (2011). Concomitant use of cholinesterase inhibitors and anticholinergics; prevelenace and outcomes. *Journal Am Geriatric Soc.*, 59(11):2069-2076.

Buerhaus P, A. D. (2009). The recent surge in nurse employment: causes and implications. *Health Aff.*, 28(4):w657-w668.

Burnard, P. E. (2000). Community mental health nurses in Wales: Self-reported stressors and coping stategies. *Journal of Psychiatric and Mental Helath Nursing*, 7,,253-528.

Burns, N. &. (2001). *The practice of nursing research (4th ed.).* Philadelphia: Saunders.

C., M. (2003). *Burnout: The Cost of Caring.* Cambridge, MA: Malor Books.

Clinic, M. (2008). *"Job burnout: Understand symptoms and take action".* Retrieved from www.mayoclinic.com/health/burnout/WL00062.

Coffey, M. (1999). Journal of Psychiatric and Mental Health Nursing. *Stress and burnout in foresnci community mental health nurses: An investigation of its causes and effects.*, 6, 433-443.

Cohen-Katz, J. S. (19(1),26-35). The effects of mindfulness-based stress reduction on nurse stress and burnout, Part II: A quantitiative and qualitative study. *Holistic Nursing Practice*, 2005.

Cohen-Katz, J. W. (2004). The effects of mindfulness-based stress reduction on nurse stress and burnout: A quantitiative and qualitative study. *Holistic Nursing Practice*, 18(6), 302-308.

Cohen-Mansfield, J. &. (2000). *Nursing staff satisfaction in long-term care.* New York: Springer Publishing Company.

Commission, T. J. (2012, January 15). *Health Care at the Crossroads.* Retrieved from Strategies for Addressing the Evolving Nursing Crisis: http://www.jointcommission.org/assets/1/18/health care at the crossroads.pdf

Cronqvist, A. B. (2001). Dissonanat imperatives in nursing: A conceptualization of stress in intensive cae in Sweden. *Intensive and Crtical Care Nursing*, 17, 228-236.

De Carl, P. (2013, November 14). *Mental health nursing: A stressful area of nursing practice? Paper presented at the Central Sydney Area Menatl Health Service Winter Symposium (Unpublished).* Retrieved from http://www.cs.nsw.gov.au/mhealth/symposium/wintsym112002.htm

Diniz BS, P. J. (2009). To treat or not to treat? A meta-analysis of the use of cholineterase inhibiots in mild cognitive impairment for delaying progression to Alzheimer's dise. *Eur Arch Psychiatry Clinal Neurosci.*, 259(4):248-256.

Ennio, C. (2010). How Much is Geriatric Caregivers Burnout Careing-Specific? *Clinical Practice & Epidemiology in Mental Helath*, 6, 66-71.

Evers, W. T. (2002). Aggressive Behvior and Burnout Among Staff of Homes for the Elderly. *International Journal of Mental Health Nursing*, 2-9.

Fagin, L. B. (1995). The Calybury community psychiatric nurse stress study: Is it more stressful to work in a hospital or the community? . *Journal of Advanced Nursing* , 22, 347-358.

Fagin, L. C. (1996). Stress, coping and burnout in mental health nurses: Findings from three reseearch studies. *The International Journal of Social Psychiatry*, 42(2),102-111.

Farrington, A. (1995). Stress and nursing. *British Journal of Nursing*, 4 574-578.

Firth, H. &. (1989). Burnout, absence and turnover amongst British nursing staff. *Journal of Occupational Psychology*, 62, 55-59.

Galantino, M. B. (2005). Association of psychological and psysiological measures of stress in health-care professionlas during an 8-wee mindfulness meditation program: Mindfulness in practice. *Stress and Healht: Journal of the Internation Society for the Investigation of Stress*, 21(4), 255-261.

George, J. (2005). *Nursing Theories: The Base for Professional Nursing Practice fith edition.* Upper Saddle River, New Jersey: Prentice Hall.

Gold, E. A. (2010). Mindfulness-based stress reduction (MBSR) for primary school teachers. *Journal of Child and Family Studies*, 19(2):184-189.

Gross, C. K. (2004). Mindfulness meditation to reduce symptoms ager organ transplant. A pilot study. *Advances in Mind-Body Medicine*, 20(2), 20-29.

Grossman, P. N. (2004). Mindfulness based stress reduction and health benefits:. *Journal of Psychosomatic Research*, 57,35-45.

Grove, W. (2006). The Role of Emotion in Rducing Burnout among Registeered Nurses. *American Sociological Association*, 50-52.

Hall, D. (2004). Work-related stress of registered nurses in hospital settings. *Journal for Nurses in Staff Development*, 20(1),6-14.

Hannigan, B. E. (2000). Burnout in communtiy mental health nurses: Findings from the all-Wales stress study. . *Journal of Psychiatric and Mntal Health Nursing*, 7,127-134.

Herbert, L. B. (2001). Annual Incidence of Alzheimer Disease in the United Staates Projected to the Years 2000 through 2050. *lzheimer Disease and Associated Disorders*, 15(4): 169-173.

Imai, H. N. (2004). Burnout and work envirnoments of public health nurses involved in mental health care. *Occupational and Environmental Medicine*, 61(9), 764-768.

Info, C. (2014, September 5). *Nurses for a Healthier Tomorrow.* Retrieved from Pscychiatric -Mental Health Nurse: http://www.nursesource.org/psychiatric.html

Invancevich, J. (2005). *Organizational Behavior and Mangement.* New York City : McGraw-Hill.

Jeanneau, M. &. (2000). Self-image and burnout in psychiatric staff. *Journal of Psychiatric and Mental Health Nursing*, 7,399-406.

Jenkin, E. (1996). Workplace homicide: Industries and occupations at high risk. *Occupational Medicine: State of the Art Reviews*, 11, 219-225.

Jenkins, R. &. (2004). Stressors, burnout and social support: Nurses in acute mental health settings. *Journal of Advanced Nursing*, 48(6), 622-631.

Kabat-Zinn, J. (1990). *Full catastrophe living: Using the wisdom of your body and mind to face stress, pain, and illness.* New York, NY: Bantam Dell.

Kabat-Zinn, J. M. (1992). Effectiveness of a meditation-based stress reduction program in the treatment of anxiety disorders. *American Journal of Psychiatry*, 149,936-943.

Kabat-Zinn, J. M. (1992). Effectiveness of a meditation-based stress reduction program in the treatment of anxiety disorders. *American Journal of Psychiatry*, 149,936-943.

Kane RL, S. T. (2007). Nursing Staffing and Quality of Patient Care. *Agency for Healthcare Research and Quality*, 151.

Keller, K. (1990). The managemnt of stress and prevention of burnout in emergency nurses. *Journal of Emergency Nursing*, 16(2), 90-95.

Kennedy, B. (2005). Stress and Burnout of Nursing Staff Working with Geriatric Clients in Long-Term Care. *Journal of Nursing Scholorship*, 37(4),381-382.

Kilfedder, C. P. (2001). Burnout in psychiatric nursing. *Journal of Advanced Nursing*, 34 (3), 383-396.

Kipping, C. (2000). Stress in mental health nursing. *International Journal of Nursing Studies*, 37,207-218.

Lachinger, H. A.-H. (2003). Workplace empowerment and magnet hosiptal characteritstics: Making the link. *Journal of Nursing Administration*, 410-422.

Lambert, V. &. (2008). Nurses' workplace stessors and coping strategies. *Indian Journal of Pallative Care*, 40-43.

Lambert, V. &. (2008). Nurses' workplace stressors and coping stratagies. *Indian Journal of Pallative Care*, 38-44.

Laschinger, H. F. (2001). Impact of structural and psycholigcal empowerment on job strain in nursing work settings: Expanding

Knater's model. *Journal of Nursing Administration*, 13(5), 260-272.

Laschinger, H. F. (2001). Impact of structural and psychological empowermanet on job strain in nursing work settings: Expanding sKanter's model. *Journal of Nursing Administration*, 13 (5), 260-272.

Lazarus, R. &. (1984). *Stress appraisal and coping.* New York: Springer.

Lazarus, R. &. (1984). *Stress Appraisal and Coping.* New York: Springer.

Lazarus, R. &. (1984). *Stress, appraisal and coping.* New York: McGraw-Hill.

Lazarus, R. (1996). *Psychological stress and the coping process.* New York:: mcGraw-Hill.

Linda H. Aiken, D. M. (2010). Implications of the California Nurse Stafing Mandate for Other States. *Health Services Research*, 45(4).

Lissa Chism, D. (2010). *The Docter of Nursing Practice.* Sudbury, Ma: Jones and Bartlett.

Mackenzie, C. P. (2006). A brief mindfulness-based stress reduction intervention for nurses and nurse aides. *Applied Nursing Research*, 19(2), 105-109.

Malugani, M. (2009, august). *Nursing Link.* Retrieved from Battling Burnout in Nurses: http://nursinglink.monster.com/benefits/articles/6239-battling-burnout-in-nursing

Marianna Virtanen, e. a. (2010, March 14). *Overtimve work and incident coronary heart disease: the Whitehall II prospective cohort study.* Retrieved from European Heart Journal: http://eurheartj.oxfordjournals.org/content, short study

Marianne Smith, M. a. (2005). Behaviors Associated with Dementia. *AJA*, 8.

Mary C. Corley, R. E. (2001). Development and Evaluation of a Moral Distess Scale. *Journal of Advanced Nursing*, (33), no. 2 250-256.

Maslach, C. &. (1981). The measurement of experienced burnout. *Jurnal of Occupational Behavior*, 2(2), 99-113.

Maslach, C. &. (1981). The measurement of experienced burnout. *Journal of Occupational Behavior*, 2,(2), 99-113.

Maslach, C. &. (1997). *The truth about burnout: How organizations cause prersonal stress and what to do about it.* . San Francisco: Jossey-Bass.

Maslach, C. (1982). *Burnout, the cost of caring.* Englewood Cliffs, NJ: Prentice Hall.

Maslach, C. (1982). *Burnout:*. New Jersey: Prentice Hall Inc.

Maslach, C. J. (1996). *Maslach Burnout Inventory Manual.* Palo Alto: Consulting Psychologists Press.

Maslach, C. J. (1996). *Maslach burnout inventory manual(3rd ed).* Mount View, CA: CPP, Inc.

Maslach, C. J. (1996). *Maslach Burnout Inventory Manual,2nd edition.* Palo Alto: Consulting Psychologist Press.

Masters, K. (2009). *Evidence -based professional nursing practice.* New York : Salibury.

McElfatrick, S. C. (2000). Assessing coping skills in mental health nurses: Is an occupational specific measure better than a gneric coping skills scale? *Personality and Individual Differences*, 28,965-976.

McShane S., &. V. (2005). *Organizational Behavior.* New York City.

Melchior, M. P.-S. (1996). The effectiveness of primary nursing on burnout among psychiatric nureses in long-stay settings. *Journal of Advanced Nursing*, 24,694-702.

Miller, L. &. (1993). *The stress solution. An action plan to manage the stress in your life.* New York: Simon & Schuster Publishing.

Moira, H. (2007). A Critical Shortage of Nurses. *Business Week*, 40-42.

Mosbey Medical Dictionary . (2009). New York: Elsierver.

Muscoft, J. &. (1998). A comparison of psychiatric nurses' and gerneral nurses' reported stress and counseling need: A case study approach. *Journal of Advanced Nursing*, 27,1317-1325.

National Institute for Health and Clincial Excellence, S. C. (2011, Noverber). *Dementia: The NICE-SCIE Guideline on Supporting People and Dementia and Their Carers in Health and Social Care.* Retrieved from National Institue for Health and Clincial Excellence : http://www.nice.org.uk/nicemedia/live/10998?30320/30320pdf

Office, G. A. (2001). *Nursing Workforce.* Retrieved from Multiple Factors Create dNurse Recruitment and Retention Problems: http://www.gao.gov/products/GAO-01-912T.

Organization, J. C. (202). *Healthcare at the Crossroads: Strategies for Addressing the Nursing Crisis.* Washington, D.C.: Joint Commission on Accrediatatin of Healthcare Organization.

Organizations, J. C. (2002). *Healthcare at the CrossRoads: Strategies for Addressing the Nursing Crisis.* Washington, D.C.

Paterson, J. J. (2010). Where do nurses go for help? A qualitative study of copoing with dealth and dying. *International Journal of Pallative Nursing*, Vol 16, 9.

Pinikahana, J. &. (2004). Stress, burnout and job satisfaction in rural psychiatric nurses: A Victorian study. *Australian Journal of Rual Health*, 120-125.

Pompili, M. R. (2006). Hopelessness and suicide risk emergeer in psychiatric nures suffering from burnout and using specific defense mecchanisms. *Archives of Psychiatric Nursing*, 20(3),135-143.

Potter, P. &. (2009). *Fundamentals of Nursing* . Boston: Salibury.

Preieb, W. J. (2004). Characteristics of teams, staff and patients: associations with outcomes of patients in asseertive outreach. *The British Journal of psychiatry*, 185:306-11.

Puntillo KA, M. J. (2006). Communication between physicians and nurses as a target for improving end-of-life care in the intensive care unit: challenges and opportunities for moving forward. *Critical Care Med.*, 332-340.

R., E. (2003). Mindful practice in action (1): Technical competence, evidence-based meicine, and relationship-centered care. *Families, Systems, & Health*, 2(1),1-9.

Raup, G. (2008). The impact of ED nurse manager leadrship style on staff nurse turnover and patient satisfaction in academic health center hospitals. *Journal of Emergency Nursing*, 34(5),403-409.

RJ., M. (2014, September 20). *Dousing Burnout.* Retrieved from http:/nurse-practisioners.advanceweb.com/Editorial/Content/Editoral aspx

RJ., N. (2014, September 20). *Dousing Burnout.* Retrieved from Http://nurse-practioners, advanceweb.com

RM., E. (2001). Just being. *West J Med.*, 174: 63-65.

Rosenstein AH, O. M. (2008). Managing disruptive physician behacior: impact on staff relationships an dpatient care. *Neurology*, 70(17):1564:1570.

Ross, M. C. (2002). Staff burnout in long-term care facilities. *Journal of the Canadian Geriatric Society*, 132-135.

Russell Doug, B. d. (2014, September 28). *Helpguide.org*. Retrieved from Dementia &Alzheimer's Care Planning and Preparing for the Road Ahead: http://ww.helpguide.org/elder/alzheimers_disease_dementias_caring_caregivers.htm

Saharain, A. F. (2008). Burnout in hospital nurses: A comparison of internal, surgery, psychiatry, and burn wards. *Internation Nursing Reveiw*, 55(1),62-67.

Salmela-Aro, K. N. (2004). The role of work -related personal projects, during two burnout interventions: a logitudinal study. *Work Stress*, 18,208-300.

Sandelowski M, &. B. (2003). Classifying the findings in qualititave studies. *Qualitative Health Research*, 13(7), 905-923.

Schaufeli, W. L. (2009). Burnout: 35 years of researcha dn practice. *Career Development International*, 14,204-220.

Schenstrom, A. R. (2006). Mindfulness-gased cognitve attitude training for primary care staff: A pilot study. *Complementary Health Practice Review*, 11(3), 144-152.

Segal, Z. W. (2002). *Mindfulness based cognitive therapy for depression.* New York: Guilford Press.

Selye, H. (1956). *The stress of life.* New York: McGraw-Hall.

Selye, H. (1974). *Stress without distress.* New York: J.B. Lippincott.

Sexton, J. T. (2000). Error, stress and teamwork in medicine and aviation: cross sectional survays. *British Medical Journal*, 320,745-749.

Shapiro, S. A. (2005). Mindfulness-based stress reduction for health care professionals: Results from a randomized trial. *International Journal of Stress Mangement*, 12(2), 164-176.

Shimizu T., M. T. (2003). Relationship between burnout and commnication skill training among Japanese hospital nurses: pilot study. *Journal of Occupational Health*, 45, 185-190.

Shirom, A. N. (2006). Overload, autonomy, and burnout as predictors of physician's quality of care. *Journal of Occupational HealthPsychology*, 11(4). 328-342.

Sitzman, K. &. (2009). *Understanding the work of nurse theorists: Acreative beginning.* Jones and Barlett Publishers.

Snelgrove, S. (1998). Occupational stress and job satisfaction: A comaprtive study of health visitors, distric nurses and community psychiatric nruses. *Journal of Nursing Management*, 6,97-104.

Sobow T, K. I. (2007). Cholinesterase inhibitiors in mild cognitive impairment; a meta-analysis of randomized controlled triails. *Neurology Neurochir Pol*, 41 (1): 13-21.

Stanks, J. (2005). *Stress at work: Mangement and prevention.* Burlington, MA: Elsevier.

(2007). *Statistical Abstract of the United States data on Alzeheimer's Disease.* Alzheimer's Association.

Statistics, U. B. (2014, September 10). *Us Bureau of Labor Statistics.* Retrieved from The Employment Situation: http://www.bls.gov/news

Stone PW. DuY, G. R. (2007). Organizational climate and occupational health outcomes in hospital nurses. *Journal Occup Environ Med.*, 49(1): 50-58.

Sullivan, P. (1993). Occupational stess in psychiatric nursing. *Journal of Advanced Nursing*, 18,591-601.

Taylor, S. (2006). *Dorthea E. Orem: Self-care deficit theory of nursing.* In: A.M.

Thomsen S, S. J. (1999). Feeling of professional fulfillment and exhaustion in mental health personnel: the importance of organisational and individual factors. *Psychother Psychosom*, 68:157-164.

Tomey, A. &. (2002). *Significance of theory for nursing as a discipline and profession. Nursing Tehorists and ther work.* St. Louis, Missouri, United States of America: Mosby.

Tophoff, J. (1999). Mindfulness training: Exploring personal change through sensory awareness. *Clinical Psycholgohy and Psychotherapy*, 6,146-155.

Tophoff, J. (2004). Mindfulness training: Exploring personal change through sensory awareness. *Constructivism in Human Science*, 8,43-54.

Tourangeau, A. &. (2009). Work stress and burnout for nurses who care for dementia patients. *Journal of Nursing*, 10-12.

Trygstaf, L. (1986). Stress and copingin psychiatric nursing. *Journal of Psychosocial Nursing*, 24,(10), 23-27.

Tully, A. (2004). Stress, sources of stess and ways of coping among psychiatric nursing students. *Journal of Psychiatric and Mental Health Nursing.*, 11, 43-47.

U.S. Department of Labor, Bureau of Labor Statistics. (2009). Retrieved from Lost-Worktime Injuries and Illnesses: Characteristics and Resulting Time Away from Work: http://www.bls.gov/news.release/osh2.nro.htm

U.S. Preventive Services Task Force (USPSTF). Screening for dementia: recommendations and rationale. (2003). Retrieved from USPSTF website: http://www.uspreventiveservicestaskforce.org/3rduspstf/dementia/dementrr.htm

Upenieks, V. (2002). Assessing differences in job differences in job satisfaction of nures in magnet and nonmagnet hospitals. *Journal of Nursing Adminstration*, 32(11),564-576.

Vahey DC, A. L. (2004). Nurse burnout and patient satisfaction. *Med Care*, 42(2).

Vahey, D. A. (2004). Nurse burnout and patient satisfaction. *Medical Care*, 42(2), II-57-II-66.

Valrie, G. M. (2004). Job Stress Among Nursing Home Certified Nursing Assistants: Comparison of Empowered and Nonempowered Work Environments. *Alzehmer's Care Quarterly*, 5,3,207-216.

Visser, M. E. (2003). Stress, satisfacrion and burnout among Dutch medical specialists. *Canadian Medical Association Journal*, 168(3),271-275.

Wheeler, H. &. (1994). Occupational stress in general nurses and midwives. *British Journal of Nursing*, 3,527-534.

Wills, M. E. (2002). *Theorectical Basess for Nursing* . Philadelphia: Lippincott Williams & wilkins.

Winstanley, J. (2000). Manchester Supervision Scale. *Nursing Standard,* 14(19),31.

Made in United States
Orlando, FL
04 November 2026

90200100R00056